Chronic Fatigue Syndrome

A Natural Healing Guide

Steve Wilkinson

Introduction by Bill Stewart

*Executive Director of the Chronic Fatigue Immune Dysfunction
Syndrome Society International, Portland, Oregon*

 Sterling Publishing Co., Inc. New York

Library of Congress Cataloging-in-Publication Data

Wilkinson, Steve.
    Chronic fatigue syndrome : a natural healing guide / Steve
Wilkinson ; introduction by Bill Stewart.
        p.   cm.
    ISBN 0-8069-7256-4
    1. Chronic fatigue syndrome.   I. Title.
RB150.F37W55   1990
616.85'28—dc20   89-48282
                                                          CIP

Copyright © 1988 by Steve Wilkinson
Published in 1990 by Sterling Publishing Co., Inc.
387 Park Avenue South, New York, New York 10016
Distributed in Canada by Sterling Publishing
c/o Canadian Manda Group, P.O. Box 920, Station U
Toronto, Ontario, Canada M8Z 5P9
Manufactured in the United States of America
All rights reserved

This book was first published in the United Kingdom in 1988 by
Thorsons Publishers Limited, Wellingborough, Northamptonshire
NN8 2RQ, England, under the title *M.E. and You: A Survivor's
Guide to Post-Viral Fatigue Syndrome*.

CONTENTS

Dedication

To Les and Gloria Wilkinson
with thanks for their constant love and support

INTRODUCTION

The phone rings at the Portland CFIDSS International office with yet another frustrated, discouraged sufferer needing desperately to know, what is this horrible thing that has altered my life? Is there any hope, and will they ever start believing what I'm saying instead of labelling me crazy? How do I find a doctor that believes me? What can I do to get better? Most callers say, "I had so much going for me; I was busy and active. I was almost never sick, and now I can barely get up to do the simplest, most necessary things."

Very few of us living in this age of modern medicine can understand why doctors are unable to find a cure for this disease, let alone understand why it is so difficult even to diagnose it. After all, aren't we geared almost from birth to believe that if something hurts, you just take a pill and it will go away? At the very least, we know that, yes, there are some things doctors can't cure, but if you are a victim of one of these incurable horrors, everyone will see you are sick and even doctors will know and acknowledge the reality of your illness. With CFS this is not usually the case: You may not look sick and all your tests may come back normal. You know you are sick and how very real your symptoms are, but doctors, friends, even family may be saying, "You just need to get going and stop being so down." Doctors may even say, "It's in your head, probably from stress, and what you need is to see a psychiatrist. Maybe that will help." You know it's not just in your head, but now you begin to doubt what you feel, what is happening. Maybe you aren't sick, but if not, why do you feel so bad? The few answers that we here at CFIDSS can give do not clear up many questions nor offer many answers, but they are the best we have.

Chronic Fatigue Syndrome is a ruthless illness, disrupting lives and families with no favored targets. It strikes young, old, rich, poor, black, white, leaving sufferers as well as families frustrated, helpless and angry. Currently there is no known cure for this syndrome; yet many people, like Steve Wilkinson, do find a road of recovery that brings them an improved quality of life as well as a return to health.

In this book Steve Wilkinson shares with us the personal story of his battle with chronic fatigue—how he worked long and hard to win the battle to reestablish himself and get back into the mainstream of life. Steve writes about symptoms such as tiredness, temperature abnormalities, fevers, infections, and depression.

He describes many forms of treatment. These include traditional medical therapies as well as holistic, naturopathic, and other alternative therapies. Aromatherapy, hydrotherapy, massage, and relaxation are only a few of the treatments Steve covers.

We here at CFIDSS International want to thank Steve Wilkinson for the effort he has made to provide information understandable to the layman and for the hope and encouragement he offers to all whose life has been affected by this debilitating illness. We encourage all who are battling this syndrome whether as a sufferer, a loved one, or a caregiver to read Steve's book. Arm yourself for the battle with the hope and encouragement that he presents in this clear, concise guide for survival. Remember, no matter how grim the circumstances may appear, we all, to some degree, have choices, and it is up to us to exercise those choices. Today's choice may be as simple as deciding that we will listen to a favorite piece of music or that we'll start reading a new book, but being able to choose even the simplest things for ourselves gives us a sense of control.

Again, we thank Steve for all he has shared with us and wish for each of you who opens this book the reward of finding your own road of recovery and improved life.

Bill Stewart, Executive Director
Chronic Fatigue Immune Dysfunction
    Society International
Portland, Oregon
October, 1989

PREFACE

Four years ago I suddenly fell ill with a mysterious and totally debilitating physical ailment that was then called Chronic Epstein-Barr Virus or CEBV, "post-viral fatigue syndrome," "Yuppie Flu," "The Hollywood Blahs," Royal Free Disease, Icelandic Disease, Neurasthenia, and Myalgic Encephalomyelitis (or M.E.), among others. In 1988 the disorder was officially recognized as Chronic Fatigue Syndrome, but the name preferred by many patients and some scientists is Chronic Fatigue Immune Dysfunction Syndrome. So today the abbreviations you are most likely to see are CFS or CFIDS in the United States, or M.E., as it is known in Canada and the United Kingdom.

Everyone argued about it. Patients argued with doctors who, for the most part, either didn't believe the disease existed at all, or believed that if it did, it was most likely an end product or symptom of some mental disturbance, and therefore the patient should be referred to a psychiatrist, with all good intentions. Patients argued with their families, friends, and co-workers, who had difficulty believing a person could look so well, yet claim to feel so bad, especially when the doctors' lab tests couldn't identify any significant abnormalities or isolate a causative agent. Doctors and top medical researchers argued about its existence as a disease, its cause, its treatments, the direction their research should take, and the meaning of their findings. Everyone argued with politicians about social security benefits, health care and insurance, and research spending.

During the first 18 months of my illness I struggled from my bed to fulfill the most basic needs, such as eating and toileting. Having spent the last 20 years of my life as an emergency-room nurse, I also explored all the traditional avenues of treatment. Then I went on to examine alternative therapies. I spent hours practising such techniques as progressive relaxation, autogenics, and biofeedback. I sought the opinions of a naturopath and a chiropractor. They offered homeopathic remedies, health food preparations, and Chinese herbs. All of these practitioners, like my M.D., could offer me treatments for my symptomatic complaints, but none could give me a cure.

I continued to explore. I was introduced to creative visualization and positive mental imagery, both a *must* for CFS patients. I developed my own form of hydrotherapy by practising those techniques in the shower, but didn't realize what I had accomplished until I read this book.

Meanwhile, Steve Wilkinson of London, England, had been dealing with CFS during the same time frame. In his book he very accurately enumerates the symptoms that CFS patients have reported and provides us with an extended list of treatments available from alternative sources. He answers the most frequently asked question we get on our CFS hotline: "What can I do to help myself?".

Here then is a comprehensive list of therapies, most of which you can practise in conjunction with your doctor's treatments. They range from massage, reflexology and aromatherapy (all of which I may try) to colonic irrigation (which I will *not*). All of these treatments have been helpful to many CFS patients, though none is assured to be effective for all of them. This is the current status of all avenues of treatment.

Steve Wilkinson's book was first released in the U.K. where it met with phenomenal success. He now offers us his easily read volume, full of insights and experience from those who have walked in our "CFS shoes." This is a true "cookbook" of alternative therapies. It shows us how we can take a personally active role in our own health process. Learn to do what you can for yourself to enhance the effects of your doctor's treatments. Those who borrow ideas from within these pages may enjoy a shortening of the course of their illness or the severity of its symptoms. Some have. If you've had CFS for very long, you probably are open to suggestions. No CFS patient should miss Steve Wilkinson's book.

Claudia Wilton Carver, R.N., C.E.N.
Board of Directors, CFIDSS International
Portland, Oregon
October, 1989

1

FROM AWARENESS
TO RECOVERY

Like many people, I gained my first awareness of CFS via the newspapers. It was being called "the Yuppie disease" and it was reported almost as a comic story. The writers took the attitude that those who had it were well-off but work-shy neurotics, and implied that the illness was a fashionable excuse for doing as little as possible. This attitude, while a tough one, was at least understandable. At that time most doctors felt the same way and were more inclined to refer their CFS patients for psychiatric treatment than accept the fact that they might have a genuine, physically based illness.

Happily, over the years I have cultivated a healthy skepticism about everything I read in the papers, and I have worked in the alternative health field long enough to know that orthodox medicine is far from having all the answers about health and well-being. When, in the course of my work, I met patients whose symptoms suggested the "Yuppie disease," I was able to approach their problem with an open mind.

It soon became clear to me that this was no imaginary

illness. By talking to as many patients as I could find, along with their families and friends, I discovered that each one experienced the same basic symptoms. If they had all been neurotic or hysterical, as the doctors tended to think, then there would not have been these widespread similarities. Also, most of the people I saw were obviously well balanced emotionally and socially, and they had all been physically and mentally healthy until the illness struck. These facts convinced me that the illness had a physical origin rather than a mental one.

Once I was satisfied in my own mind that the illness was organic, and not evidence of some psychosomatic disorder, I began to explore various methods of treatment. The patients I had contacted during my investigations were happy to try alternative therapies because there was then, and is now, no definitive orthodox treatment. With my encouragement and advice they experimented with different therapies, and almost all of them found a treatment that helped them to live and work as normal.

Then, as other projects came up and the emphasis of my work altered, I gradually lost touch with the Yuppie disease and these patients. By this time the newspapers had started calling it "post-viral fatigue syndrome," and were reporting it as a serious illness. This new respect from the media came about because evidence that the illness had a physical cause was growing fast as more doctors and scientists were looking into it.

In the spring of the following year I caught a nasty low-grade flu virus, and spent a couple of weeks feeling miserable. With the perfect vision of hindsight, I now know that this was probably the first intrusion of the CFS virus into my system. At the time, it did not occur to me to consider it as anything more than flu. I soon discovered my mistake.

During the following weeks and months I was constantly ill, with a baffling array of symptoms. The most annoying of these was a violent, angry rash that appeared on any part of my body exposed to the sun. The rash was ferociously itchy and grew steadily worse. From small red pin-pricks it developed into large swollen bumps that split and cracked. My doctor told me it was prickly heat, a rash caused by the salt in sweat irritating the skin as the sweat evaporates. This surprised me since most of the time I was feeling extremely cold; I spent much of the summer bundled up in sweaters in an effort to keep warm. I simply was not sweating to any noticeable degree. Also, I was weak and tired the whole time, and frequently confused and depressed. It seemed rather optimistic to assume that prickly heat could account for all of these symptoms. Eventually, because the broken skin became infected, I was given antibiotics. These helped, but the rash persisted throughout the rest of the summer and fall.

For a few weeks in November, everything seemed fine and I started to feel that life was returning to normal. Then, without any warning, I became severely ill. I constantly felt exhausted and deeply depressed. Weakness of the muscles and the will prevented me from doing even the simplest things for myself. I was always in pain and cold and shivery, but at night fevers struck and my sweat soaked the bed-clothes. I could not speak properly, or understand anything I saw or heard. My joints and muscles were continuously sore and stiff, and the pains in my head, neck and nerves defied description. I fell into an uneasy sleep every few hours, awakening unrefreshed. I felt sick at the thought of food and lost weight rapidly. I lost the use of my memory, often stopping dead in the middle of a sentence, forgetting what I was about to say. To complicate matters, the glands in my neck became infected and I suffered badly from urethritis. I was in a dreadful state.

At this point my doctors declared that I was suffering from glandular fever. This seems an odd diagnosis now, but then I simply could not think clearly enough to understand what they were saying or to question their opinion. I went along with what they said, hoping desperately to get well. Unfortunately, I got worse instead of better.

I suffered throughout the next year, especially in summer when the rash returned to add to the other difficulties. The doctors continued to treat me for glandular fever, even though three separate blood tests showed that I did not have that disease. The only treatment that had any effect whatsoever was antibiotics—I ended up taking these for over 20 weeks during that terrible year. But I certainly wouldn't recommend this since there is substantial evidence that antibiotics exacerbate CFS and this can be very damaging in the long run.

Just as I started to think that I was never going to get well, the illness began to recede. For the first time in months I could do things for myself and take an interest in my surroundings. Most glorious of all was the fact that I could think again—I had a brain instead of wet cotton wool. I soon found out, though, that I had to be extremely careful. The slightest mental or physical exertion left me feeling awful. As soon as I became strong enough, I searched out all my reference books and put my newly refound brain into gear for a good hard think about what had been happening to me.

One thing was immediately obvious. I did not have glandular fever. With that out of my mind, I started to look through my notes and references to figure out exactly what had been wrong. Of course, it soon became clear that I was suffering from a classic case of "post-viral fatigue syndrome," as it was then called. As I read back through my notes on the subject and on my interviews with patients, it was like reading a list of my own symptoms.

It was comforting to be able to put a label on my illness. It immediately became less frightening, less ominous. At the same time, it made me face up to a few hard facts: At that time no one knew what caused the illness; there was no treatment for it; and there was not even a suggestion of a cure. However, I knew from past experience that alternative therapies could help, and that sufferers could live and work largely as normal if they were sensible. Cheered by the prospect of being able to help myself, I started sorting out those therapies that seemed most suitable for me.

Begging help from friends and colleagues—masseurs, herbalists, reflexologists, healers and so on—and putting my own skills to use, I started to try the various therapies. It was a long process. Some treatments were obviously unsuitable and could be ruled out at once. Others were borderline, but I felt I had to try them to see if they could be helpful. Along the way there were periods of weeks, sometimes months, when the illness returned and I felt myself slipping back to square one. These were perhaps the worst times of all. It seemed as though I was losing all hope as well as my fragile grasp on health. But as I sorted through the therapies and continued regularly with those that offered the most promise, a wonderful thing started to happen. The relapses became shorter and less frequent. As the periods between bouts of illness grew longer, I grew stronger. I started to believe that the therapies I had selected were eventually going to prove effective. At last I felt as though it was possible to win.

One evening my father told me about a radio program he had been listening to. It was a medical phone-in during which a caller had described symptoms that were exactly the same as mine. The radio doctor had advised her to contact the M.E. Association. (CFS is known as Myalgic Encephalomyelitis—or M.E.—in the U.K. and in Canada.) As I had never heard of this group, I wrote to them to find out about it. In due course they sent me some leaflets that described how the illness had been known as post-viral fatigue syndrome, and that now it had been reclassified "myalgic encephalomyelitis." Most important of all, they said that researchers had identified the Epstein-Barr virus as the potential cause of the disease, and could now test for its presence.

I was fairly ill at this time and seeing my doctor regularly. At my next appointment I brought up the subject of M.E. and asked for a test. The response astounded me. The doctor obviously knew nothing about myalgic encephalomyelitis, which was unfortunate but understandable. However, her attitude was that if she knew nothing about the illness, then I couldn't possibly be suffering from it. I was feeling too ill and weak to argue, but then and there I made up my mind to find a more sympathetic doctor.

Luckily I found one fairly soon. The new doctor's practice was miles away from where I lived, but the difficulties of the journey were made worthwhile when I got there. He was charming and courteous, and willing to listen to me as I described what I had been going through and explained what I thought might be the cause. He then examined me thoroughly and took several blood samples for analysis. He explained that though he thought I had M.E. he would test for several other possibilities at the same time. Greatly reassured, I left with high hopes. Two weeks later he phoned me with the test results and confirmed the presence of the Epstein-Barr antibodies in my blood sample.

Even though I had been sure that this was my problem, the relief of knowing definitely was incredible. With renewed strength I returned to my therapies. I was determined to get the virus out of my system, or at least to learn how to keep it under control.

My confidence in the therapies was well founded. For months now I have been free of all major symptoms for the first time since the illness started. When I think back to how ill I was, this seems an unbelievable achievement, and even now every day brings another small improvement. There are still relapses—times of weakness and tiredness—but these can be controlled and they pass quickly. Thankfully, I am once again able to work and play with the energy and enthusiasm that I believed had gone forever.

My story of illness and diagnosis is not at all unusual. Since finding my way back to health I have met many other people who have experienced the same thing. Many of them have terrible tales to tell, not only about the physical and mental problems caused by the illness, but also about their difficulties with the medical establishment. I have met children whom the authorities wanted to label "phobic" or "educationally subnormal" because of their illness. I don't like to think about the numbers of children who may have received an inaccurate diagnosis. For them, psychiatric treatment could be mistreatment.

Adults, too, have been wrongly diagnosed in all sorts of painful and humiliating ways. A large number, particularly women, are told by their doctors that they are neurotic, menopausal, hysterical, or emotionally unbalanced. Some are then pressured into accepting anti-depressants and other drugs. I cannot emphasize too strongly how damaging this can be. We can only hope that now that more is known about the disease, more GPs will come to understand it and deal with their patients properly.

In the meantime, we need to develop a slightly wary attitude towards the medical establishment. Those of you who think that you may have the illness, and those who have just been diagnosed, should learn a vital lesson from all of us who have been through it: Your doctor should be your friend. By this I mean simply that your doctor should be someone you can relate to easily, and someone whom you feel is on your side, willing to be supportive and concerned enough to help you find suitable treatment. A doctor who is ignorant about the disease, skeptical about your problems or unwilling to seek out solutions is no help at all. If your doctor is unsympathetic, don't be afraid to ask for a second opinion or to be referred to a specialist. In any case, get in touch with one of the CFS support groups. They probably know of patients in your area who have already been through these problems and have found a sympathetic doctor.

Having drawn attention to the problem of finding a helpful medical advisor, I would also like to make you aware of your responsibility toward the doctor you have found. People like myself, whose symptoms include intense mental disorientation and lack of comprehension, can create problems for doctors. It is vital that your physicians get a clear picture of exactly what is happening to you. If you cannot understand the doctors' questions, cannot remember what has been happening to you or cannot speak coherently, you will not be able to give your advisors all the information about your symptoms that they need. If this happens, your doctors will be making decisions based on only a partial knowledge of your situation. Obviously, this reduces your changes of being helped, so you must find some other way to communicate effectively.

Many times in the early days of my illness I arrived at the doctor's office or the hospital in a state of total confusion. I could not understand anything I saw or heard. I could not remember clearly; I could not speak without slurring and mumbling. In short, I was in no way able to communicate the complex range of ailments and symptoms that had taken over my life.

In my more lucid moments, I realized that this was a ridiculous waste of time for everyone concerned. I could not expect to get any help unless I could state my problems reasonably clearly. So I got into the habit of keeping a notepad lying around. On this pad I would jot down my symptoms and when they occurred. In this way I always had up-to-date information about my state of health. Just before every appointment I could read through the list to refresh my memory, or, if I was particularly ill, I could simply hand the notes to the doctor when I arrived. During the times when I was too ill to write, I would ask a friend to make the notes for me.

Keeping notes like this might seem an incredible chore when you are ill, but it is a very effective way to make sure that your doctor fully understands what is happening to you. Alternatively, if you share a house with friends or family, you could ask them to describe your situation to the doctor for you, making sure that they include even the minor symptoms. However you decide to do it, you must be certain that you communicate fully and properly with your physician. This is the only way in which you can improve your chances of prompt and correct diagnosis and support.

The importance of a correct diagnosis cannot be overstated. All the time you are in doubt about the cause of your illness, you are fighting against an invisible enemy, never knowing how, when or where it might strike next. This leaves you in a constant state of doubt and fear. The uncertainty about what is happening to your body can be intensely stressful. It is all too easy to imagine that you have a brain tumor or something equally frightening when you are continually confused and in pain. Even if you consciously know that these worries are ridiculous, at lower levels your mind remains restless and anxious. As soon as you get a positive diagnosis, your fears are put to rest and the energy tied up in worrying is free to help you overcome the illness. For people who have been sick for a long time, finally getting a positive diagnosis produces a feeling of relief and well-being that borders on euphoria.

This is strange when you consider that a diagnosis of CFS often amounts to a sentence of years of pain and difficulty. In my experience, the relief stems from the fact that the enemy has become visible. At last you know exactly what it is that you are up against. You know that the disease is not fatal, and that is it not degenerative. Knowing that you will not die from CFS, you can start devoting all your energy to learning to live with it. And this is the first step toward conquering your illness.

Living with CFS is an exercise in the fine art of self-awareness. Gradually, you learn about your own tolerances and limitations: how much you can do without suffering for it later; how long you can concentrate; how late you can stay up; how early you can rise; how much you can work, or play, or write, or talk, or watch TV, or drink, or think, or listen, or walk, or read, or eat, or . . . or . . . or . . . All of these things, which you used to take for granted, suddenly have to be measured and carefully considered. You need to remain constantly aware of your resources of strength and take very good care that you do not exhaust them.

Of course, your limitations will be completely different from everyone else's. You will find that your tolerance for some things is much greater than for others. For example, like many patients, I suffered badly in the middle of the night. I would wake up with a high fever, dripping with sweat, in great pain and mental confusion. Unable to sleep again, my mind would spiral into the pain, depression would set in, and I would spend the rest of the night in utter misery—feeling too weak and sick even to cry. This happened every night for months. I desperately needed something to occupy me during those long, lonely nights. My tolerance for books, magazines and TV was absolutely nil— I could not understand a single thing—but I found that I could tolerate playing cards. This began a habit that has persisted to this very day. For some reason my mind could take in and make sense of the thousands of games of solitaire. I played during a period when everything else was completely beyond me.

Having discovered this, I had a weapon to help fight the loneliness and misery of those dark nights. I no longer felt so helpless and hopeless, which was a great step forward. Instead of fearing the nights, I knew that I could get through them with a minimum of suffering.

Of course, the next step was to exploit this tolerance for all it was worth. I asked friends to go to the library and bring me books on solitaire, so that I had a wide range of games to suit my mental states—some demanding, others less so. I played the simple games when I was ill, and the small triumph of winning helped keep me cheerful and optimistic. During convalescent phases, when my mind became more agile and responsive, I played the most demanding games to fend off boredom and frustration.

In playing cards I had found an occupation to help focus my mind outside myself, away from the illness. This provided valuable breathing spaces in each day when I forgot, as much as possible, the pain and weakness that afflicted me the rest of the time. Without this, every day would have been totally dominated by illness.

Other people have found different ways of achieving these breathing spaces. One woman I know found that she could tolerate making simple flower arrangements when she was too ill to do anything else, so she spent sleepless nights arranging and rearranging pretty decorations for her friends and her home. During periods of mental alertness, she read books about Japanese arrangements and began to experiment with new shapes, colors and combinations. In the same way that I now keep a deck of cards around the house, she keeps a few bunches of dried flowers in the closet as insurance against those bad days and nights that crop up every now and again.

Anything that is physically undemanding and sufficiently stimulating to interest the mind will help you get into your own breathing space and away from your problems for a short while. The benefits of this cannot be overestimated. It allows you to realize that life does exist outside your illness and that you can do something competently, even if it is only playing cards against yourself. Mentally and emotionally it gives you something to hold on to, and it keeps you from losing all self-respect and all expectation of health. Most important of all, it provides a little relief from your constant awareness of a heavy, painful body and a confused, unhappy mind.

Learning about the breathing spaces was an important development in my approach to the illness, and the relief the spaces provided helped me to concentrate more fully on the therapies that were proving successful. This book is all about the breathing spaces that can be found in therapies themselves, and it is written with the aim of helping every individual find a safe, simple treatment that will provide relief.

Most of the therapies in this book are suitable for the individual to use at home, but some require the assistance of a professional practitioner. In every case, people who suffer from CFS have found the treatment successful. The therapies explained and recommended here have all been approved by other patients and are known to be effective. From this short list of treatments you can select the ones that work for you.

Before examining the therapies in greater detail, let's take a closer look at the illness. Making the enemy fully visible will help you to replace uncertainty with an understanding of exactly what is happening inside your own body. Understanding what the disease can do will help you to defend yourself against it with greater success.

2

THE DISEASE . . .

CFS may be caused by a virus—perhaps one of the 80 or more viruses known collectively as the "entero" virus group, which enter the body through the digestive system and affect the brain, nerves and muscles. Or, it may be caused by a herpes virus, such as the suspect Epstein-Barr virus—or possibly even by an unknown retrovirus. It could even be caused by something totally new. Very little is known for sure. Since the Epstein-Barr virus was discovered, an immense effort has been made by researchers to find out the full story of this elusive germ. It is now generally recognized that the Epstein-Barr virus does not in fact cause the disease, and its role remains uncertain. As yet, no major breakthroughs have taken place, but gradually small pieces of the puzzle are falling into place. There is generally a feeling of optimism and the sense that we shall soon understand the causes of this illness more fully.

CFS may have been around for a very long time. Outbreaks of what appeared to be CFS varying severity have occurred all over the world and until recently no one could explain what caused the malady. In 1955 an illness at the

Royal Free Hospital in London affected doctors and nurses, bringing their work to a grinding halt. The "Royal Free disease," as it was called, was said to have been caused by mass hysteria, which is one of those explanations that really explains nothing. None of the doctors who suggested it could define what mass hysteria was, or how it worked or why it should affect doctors and nurses but not patients. Nevertheless, mass hysteria became the official explanation for the events at the Royal Free.

An outbreak in Iceland, which affected most of the inhabitants of a small town, received much the same reception. Newspapers reported the medical authorities as saying that the mass hysteria was to blame for the townspeople's illness. The illness itself was unimaginatively referred to as "Icelandic disease." The mass hysteria theory lent a semblance of scientific credibility to the notion that CFS patients were mentally unstable. It has taken many years for the medical establishment to realize and admit that they may have been seriously mistaken, but even now many doctors are unaware of the true nature of CFS. Some doctors who believed CFS to be a psychosomatic disorder are reluctant to face up to proof that the disease may result from a viral infection. Some GPs still assess us as malingerers or hysterics and tell us to "pull ourselves together." Fortunately, many doctors are more understanding than this and make an effort to keep up with recent developments in research. They are willing to acknowledge that their patients are suffering from a debilitating disorder and offer valuable support and advice. Hopefully, before much longer, all doctors will adopt this more sensible and sensitive approach.

The Hows And Whys of CFS

Meanwhile, we are left with many unanswered questions about the illness. For example, we do not know how people catch it. Although there is no firm evidence to prove the case one way or another, it seems unlikely that it is transmitted from person to person. If this is correct, then the causative àgent must exist and possibly multiply somewhere in the environment. This, of course, would explain how large groups of people could catch it at the same time, as happened in Iceland, at the Royal Free Hospital and, more recently, at a school in Scotland where the entire staff contracted a similar illness.

Another important question concerns the duration of the illness. Again, no firm evidence is available one way or the other, but various authorities are suggesting that it lasts for two years, five years, ten years or even indefinitely. As there is such a disparity among the various estimates, none of them can be taken seriously. I suggest that you ignore all of them and concentrate on getting well in the shortest possible time.

It should not be long before researchers fully understand the hows and whys of CFS, but until they do we must resign ourselves to being in the dark about it. However, even without scientific evidence, we can gather much useful information by going directly to people who have the illness and finding out how it affects them. Having talked to many patients, I find that there is a pattern to the illness that is more or less the same in most cases. Understanding this pattern helps people to know what to expect, and being forewarned in this way can prevent a lot of pain and worry.

The Basic Pattern

The first sign of CFS may come after a viral infection of some kind, quite often a form of gastric flu—sometimes with respiratory complications—that takes longer than usual to clear up. Though the symptoms of the infection gradually disappear, the patient is left with the symptoms of CFS: extreme tiredness, fatigue, coldness, etc. Very often people assume that the problem is just the aftereffects of the flu or whatever they had. It's only when it gets more severe and continues for weeks or months that they start to think that something else may be wrong.

This first stage of the illness is very important. Assuming that their symptoms are just the aftereffects of the virus, most people return to a normal lifestyle and try to work through the weakness. This is a serious mistake. Forcing yourself to work, even if it is only doing minor things like dusting and shopping, can intensify all the symptoms and prolong the illness. If you really push yourself hard to get things done, it can prompt your symptoms to degenerate into a chronic state. If you have had such an infection and for any reason suspect that instead of the normal convalescent weakness you have CFS, see your doctor at once and ask for an evaluation and workup.

The symptoms of CFS are a lot like normal convalescent weakness. When you are getting over the flu, for example, you feel tired, weak and shaky; and simple tasks require more effort than normal. CFS patients suffer all of these symptoms constantly and in an extreme form, but often they have muscular pain and swelling, back and head pain and extreme coldness as well. Other obvious symptoms are severe memory lapses, lack of comprehension and rapid mood swings.

For some, the illness will continue exactly as it started for a lengthy period, sometimes for years. For most of us it is a different story. The illness continues for a period of weeks or months (often not more than eight months); then the patient starts to improve. Day by day the symptoms recede and the patient starts to feel human again. This convalescent period is wonderful, but it is a time to take great care because all is not as it seems to be. Although you feel stronger, you are still not strong. Many patients, fooled by the improvement, assume that they are recovering and start to live a more strenuous life. As soon as they attempt things that are too much for them, the illness returns with speed and force.

CFS patients soon learn that to give themselves the best chance of health they need to remain constantly aware of their energy levels and never tire themselves to the point where the illness can take over again. This can impose strict limitations on a lifestyle. Some people can work only part-time, if at all. Others have to be sure to get to bed early every night. Some must rest in the afternoon or after exercise. It's difficult to adjust to the fact that the illness is always in the background, ready to surface again if you give it the slightest chance. If you do not adjust to this new fact of life, you will probably suffer relapse after relapse. Fighting the illness by making an extra effort to get things done is a natural but very foolish response. Paradoxically, the only way to beat the condition is to give in to it. Rest and relaxation are the only sure ways to relieve the symptoms and prevent continual attacks.

You can extend the periods of convalescence and relatively good health following bouts of illness through cautious and sensible living. But even this does not necessarily prevent relapses. Many people have found that the illness has a cycle, so that at various times of the year they are prone to relapse no matter how careful they are. A common pattern is to relapse in the fall or winter and recover in the spring.

Relapses, whether they stem from over-exertion or natural causes, tend to be as bad or worse than previous bouts. For many people the first bout of illness is the weakest, and in each subsequent bout the illness gets stronger and takes longer to recover from. This pattern of gradual degeneration is very common, but in most cases it eventually halts of its own accord. At this point you may still have relapses, but they will be no worse than the preceding ones. Unfortunately, this is often because they *can* get no worse—you have become as ill as you can get.

So, usually the illness seems to follow a pattern of bouts and remissions. Their length will vary from person to person, and also from time to time in the same individual. Many things can trigger relapses, but in all cases mental or physical over-exertion is a major cause. When you are in a bout of illness, something as simple as making a cup of tea can amount to over-exertion, so you have to be very careful.

The Psychological Component

Although it has now been proved that CFS is an illness with an organic cause, it seems to me and to others that there is a strong psychological component that should not be overlooked. Everyday experience shows us that our feelings have a strong effect on everything we do. When you are in a state of sadness or depression you feel slow and heavy, and living is a constant struggle. Conversely, when you feel happy and outgoing you seem to have a steady flow of energy at your fingertips. This is a simple example of the way in which moods can color, or even control, our physical strength and stamina. With CFS exactly the same is true, and to a heightened degree. Whether this is because of interference produced by the organism's effect on the emotional centers of the brain, or whether it simply happens because physical weakness allows the emotional influence to become dominant, we don't know. Nevertheless, it is a very real effect.

One woman I know had been in a remission period for almost a year. She had achieved it by using alternative therapies and generally taking a sensible approach to life. She had returned to work full-time and felt that she was in control of the illness. One day, without any warning, she began to experience strong pain in her leg muscles. These muscles were where she had been affected most severely during the worst of her illness. Realizing that she had obviously done something wrong and allowed the illness to creep up on her, she tried to figure out what her mistake had been. She checked the amounts of exercise she had taken, made sure her diet had been good, and thought about whether she'd been losing any sleep. Everything in these areas was fine, so she was at a loss as to what had gone wrong.

This woman was in one of the caring services, and during the week before her problem she had dealt with some cases that had upset her badly. Once she realized that it was the emotional turmoil that had triggered the leg pain, she dealt with it quickly and effectively by talking out her feelings and removing the emotional burden. She immediately felt better and has had no more pain since. This is an important lesson for all CFS sufferers. Your mental and emotional energies are just as important as your physical ones and must be protected in the same way.

When you are constantly cold, tired and in pain, "listening" to your body becomes almost second nature. You are aware of how you are feeling from moment to moment, often uncomfortably so, and you immediately know when your body starts telling you that you have done enough or too much. This is practically a built-in instinct, so it is fairly simple to bring it into full conscious awareness. It is not nearly so simple to "listen" to your feelings. Many of us go through life carrying a heavy load of unhappiness, fear, doubt, insecurity or anger of which we are hardly conscious. This load has a negative effect on us mentally and physically, but when we are healthy, we can overlook or ignore it easily. When we have CFS, the load suddenly becomes intolerable. It puts stress on our systems, causes an immediate and dramatic worsening of all symptoms, and can create greater long-term difficulties unless it is removed. Talking to someone who is understanding and sympathetic is the best cure for these inner difficulties, but self-awareness and the inner therapies mentioned later in this book are even better because they prevent stress from arising in the first place.

Just as anything that intensifies your emotions—making you feel down, uncomfortable or uptight—complicates the illness, physical stress is harmful too. Anything that makes you feel tense should be strictly avoided while you're in a bout of illness, and only experienced to a reasonable extent when you're in remission. Physical tension is the outward sign of inner stress and discomfort, so by avoiding things and situations that cause physical tension you'll be relieving the burden on your inner self, too.

One of the things I have always found stressful is travelling by public transportation. I avoid buses completely and only take trains when there is no practical alternative. Train trips leave me feeling very uptight, particularly during the rush hour. The physical tension it produces is the outward echo of inner stress caused by an intense dislike of being confined in a small space with other people.

When I'm feeling fit I can cope with the effects of this stress, but since CFS, train travel wipes out all my resources for the rest of the day. I soon came to realize that I had a simple choice. I could either waste my mental and physical energy on a stressful pursuit, leaving myself drained and prone to illness, or I could use my resources to feel well and happy and achieve something worthwhile. It was not difficult to decide between the two. I have adjusted my lifestyle to eliminate this activity as much as possible.

A Positive Change

Unfortunately, having CFS is not a simple business. It's not a case of being ill, getting well and then living life as before. If you wish to reduce the illness to manageable proportions and make the best use of your time and energy, you are forced to make changes. Some of these changes are simple, outward ones: Altering your routine, using alternative therapies regularly, allowing for your illness where you cannot work around it. Other changes are more complex, having to do with your inner world. Learning to "listen" to your emotions is the first and most important of these, and this can lead to a change in attitudes, beliefs and expectations.

One patient I knew, when talking about the illness, said, "It's been awful, but in a way it has been good, too. I have found out so much about myself that I never knew before. I am more capable of living a happy life now than I ever was before I got sick." I think that this is a wonderful attitude and agree with it wholeheartedly. Even though you set out to make your life better by understanding the disease, you end up making a happier life for yourself by understanding yourself in a way you never could have before. Along the way you can lose all sorts of negative feelings and gain a full knowledge of what is important to you. When you regain your health you may find that you have new and positive attitudes about many things in your life.

Having examined the overall pattern of illness, let's look more closely at the day-to-day effect it has on your body— the symptoms.

3

. . . AND ITS SYMPTOMS

Part of the reason why CFS was thought to be a psycho-somatic disorder for so long is that different patients re-ported different symptoms. One might complain of coldness and headaches, while another sought help for fe-vers and leg pain. Before the Epstein-Barr virus (EBV) was associated with the disorder, there was little reason to as-sume that these two people were experiencing the same disease. However, what was overlooked for a long time was the fact that only major symptoms were taken into account when a diagnosis was attempted. Once minor symptoms were also considered, a pattern emerged that linked almost all CFS patients.

CFS can produce a vast range of symptoms, affecting all parts of the body. In a few people, one symptom is dominant and the others absent or slight enough to cause no concern. In the vast majority of cases, however, a group of dominant symptoms are complicated by minor problems of many dif-ferent types. By noting all of them, major and minor, you develop a list of symptoms that is familiar to all patients. What varies is the severity of each symptom. Every patient experiences a unique combination of affects, but the same symptoms occur in most cases.

This difference in symptoms complicates the matter of treatment. As there is no overall cure, therapists can only hope to treat individual symptoms successfully as they arise. This means that the therapy that works for one person may have little or no effect upon another. Also, because the minor symptoms can change from day to day, or even from hour to hour, it is difficult to develop a course of treatment that is consistently effective. You always need to keep a weather-eye on your symptoms and stay alert to changes. In this way you'll always know which of the symptoms are your major priority for treatment. Use the following section to help you decide which problems are your priorities and concentrate on treating these first. Once you have achieved some relief, you can experiment to find successful ways of dealing with the minor symptoms.

If you have just been diagnosed as having CFS, some of the symptoms here may be new to you. Don't worry. Not every patient experiences every symptom. Your pattern of illness is probably already established, so if you have not had a particular symptom already, you may not get it. Your major symptoms will only change slowly, if at all.

If you're wondering whether or not you have CFS, use the following section as a guide. If you have experienced several or many of the symptoms over a long period of time, contact your doctor and request a blood test for EBV and a complete diagnostic workup. If you have had severe trouble with one or more symptoms, it's important to see your doctor. Don't forget that there may be other causes for all the individual symptoms, and many of the other illnesses are easier to treat than CFS. Even if you do eventually receive a confirmed diagnosis of CFS, don't be disheartened. The sooner you find out, the sooner you can learn to live with the illness and find an effective remedy.

THE PHYSICAL SYMPTOMS

TIREDNESS

I'm putting this symptom first because I have found that it is perhaps the most common one. Very few are lucky enough to escape problems in this area. Like all the symptoms, it can vary enormously in its severity, so I shall try to illustrate the full spectrum of its influence.

Tiredness was one of my own first symptoms, and has been one of the longest lasting. In its strongest form, it can totally disrupt your lifestyle because in every waking moment you have an intense yearning to sleep. When sitting or lying down, there is no way in which you can stop your eyes from closing. When moving around, your only thought is of a chair or bed. You constantly feel as though you have been up all night at a particularly energetic party. Even though you sleep as much as sixteen hours a day, you wake up feeling totally unrefreshed and want to go straight back to bed.

In its milder form, the fatigue is like the aftereffects of flu. You feel relatively strong first thing in the morning, but by the afternoon your strength is at an end. Afternoon naps and early nights are very appealing, and they are also a very sensible way to treat this symptom. You feel slightly below par most of the time, as though you hadn't had enough sleep the previous night. Even so, you will probably find yourself sleeping much more than normal.

At best, the tiredness becomes a minor inconvenience. You may have to buy a louder alarm clock to make sure that you get up in the morning, and you will probably find that by mid- to late afternoon you are feeling low. I always have a low period between four and six p.m. To allow for this, I make sure that nothing too energetic or demanding is scheduled for this period when I am at my weakest. By early evening I have picked up again and feel reasonably alert until bedtime, which I make sure is at a reasonable hour. This pattern of highs and lows is very common in periods of convalescence and remission.

During the worst stages of fatigue there is little that you can do to help yourself except give in to the demand for sleep and more sleep. Some sufferers report that doctor-prescribed stimulants can help, but the majority find that they should be avoided. The best treatment for fatigue in its mildest form is to use self-awareness and will power: Be aware of your low periods during the day and work around them, establishing a regular routine that you can keep to. The midway form will respond well to the various treatments I'll outline later.

WEAKNESS

This is also a widespread symptom and it is most often experienced together with tiredness.

Muscular weakness is one of the most frustrating symptoms. Even if you are feeling all right otherwise, this weakness can prevent you from doing anything. When it is at its worst, simple actions like standing, sitting and lifting light objects become extremely difficult, and walking can be close to impossible. Some sufferers have been confined to bed or a wheelchair during chronic phases.

Usually, however, weakness is not so severe. In the more common milder form, the lack of physical strength makes life difficult in any number of small ways. Making a cup of tea seems to require the effort more often associated with climbing Everest. Bottles and jars have to be opened by a helpful friend. Faucets cannot be turned on and off, heavy pots and pans cannot be used and even heavy clothing can sometimes present problems. Anything requiring muscular effort becomes immensely difficult. At this stage beware of exercise of any sort. Frustration can make you attempt to do things that are too strenuous. The result will often be a relapse into greater weakness, and if you do too much exercise, you can provoke the symptom into becoming chronic.

As with tiredness, the mildest form of weakness is simply a scaled-down version of the intense symptom. You feel that your muscles do not have the strength and resilience that they should have. Like tiredness, this symptom is best treated with self-awareness and will power. Arrange your days so that you undertake the more strenuous activities when you're at your strongest, and do as little as possible during your low periods. Once you've established a good routine, stick to it with every ounce of will power you possess. Don't be tempted to do spring cleaning or go out with friends when you know you should rest.

Many people have found muscle weakness a very sensitive symptom to deal with. It gives you a clear indication of your current reserves of strength, and if you overstep them, you will suffer for it in the days or weeks to come. You can treat weakness with any relaxation-based therapy. Acupuncture, acupressure, reflexology and hypnotism have also been effective. On a preventive basis, be sure that your diet includes plenty of energy-giving foods.

PAIN

The bad news is that this illness can cause intense pain in any part of the body. The good news is that no sufferers seem to have pain all over, all of the time. You may find that you have difficulties in one particular area and are free of pain elsewhere.

The most common pain is in the head, neck and/or back. It is similar to a migraine headache: continuous sharp bursts that seem to echo around your skull and down your spine, often accompanied by extreme light sensitivity and nausea. Unfortunately, there is little that can be done to help, and the headaches can continue for long periods. Relaxation is the therapy that brings most relief in the long run, with pain-killers used when necessary to provide short-term relief. It's a good idea to try different kinds of pain-killers. I have found that some brands work better for me than others. Those containing Ibuprofen help me most, and when I recommend these brand to others, they are usually pleased by their effectiveness.

As well as having the migraine-type headaches, you may find that you are more prone to the normal kind. These center around the eyes and thump away endlessly. Sometimes they fade into the background and disappear, but often the only thing that will stop them is a good night's sleep.

Muscular pain is common and is not always associated with other muscular problems. At worst, your muscles grow sensitive to pressure and the lightest touch can be extremely painful. This happens particularly in the long muscles of the arms and legs. They can also feel hard to the touch, and severe swelling can develop. In this case, avoid all exercise if possible. In its weaker form, muscular pain is a continuous dull ache that escalates to a burning sensation if you exercise too much.

Nerve pain is usually mild—a tingling, twitching or irritated sensation just below the surface of the skin. Occasionally, people complain about it escalating to a neuralgia-type pain, but this is relatively uncommon.

Joint and bone pain is extremely hard to describe. When you have it, you feel as though your bones are sore and tired—worn out, in fact. I have never come across a severe case of this type of pain, but it is frequently an unpleasant undercurrent to other symptoms. It usually centers in the spine, arms or hands.

Chest pain is one of the most frightening symptoms. Many people have thought they were having a heart attack when this problem struck. The pain comes in stabs and bursts and seems to center around the heart. It can be accompanied by palpitations or missed heartbeats. The pain is aggravated by quick breathing or by rapid chest movements—the kind that happen when you laugh—and it can be triggered by either. The pain will pass quickly if you sit quietly, relax and breathe slowly and deeply for a few minutes. Obviously, if you have any history of heart problems or are in a high-risk group, check with your doctor immediately.

TREMORS

People who have not experienced this symptom seem to consider it a minor thing, but in practice it is an embarrassing and awkward problem. The muscles of the arms and legs, particularly the hands and feet, twitch continuously, so that there is a constant shaking and quivering of the affected part of the body. It is not painful, but it can prevent you from walking properly or carrying anything. Even if only the extremities are shaking, it is intensely irritating if it continues for a while. It also makes you seem clumsy because you keep spilling drinks or tripping over your own feet. The relaxation-based therapies, biochemical remedies and homeopathy can all help with this symptom.

TEMPERATURE

There are many temperature abnormalities, but by far the most common is coldness. This can take the form of cold hands and feet or a general all-over chilliness, or it can vary according to your other symptoms—the more your muscles ache, the colder you become, for example. At its worst it becomes very intense, and you shiver no matter how high the thermostat is set or how many warm clothes you wear. At this level, coldness is accompanied by a worsening of all other symptoms, and perhaps it is caused by this worsening. There is no escaping it, but long hot baths can relieve the situation for reasonable periods. Many people find that their temperature is consistently below normal by a degree or more, even when they are feeling relatively healthy.

Sudden increases in temperature can also occur after any exertion, and this usually happens after a meal. If you take small amounts of food fairly often, this can help you maintain a reasonable body temperature.

FEVERS

Intense fevers can occur when the illness is at its worst, and I certainly experienced them, but more often they are low grade fevers with body temperature rising to no more than 100°F. My fevers usually struck at night, and if you happen to be awake when one starts, you can feel your temperature rising minute by minute. If you are asleep during the onset, as is usually the case, the first thing you become aware of as you wake from the extreme heat is sweat—and plenty of it. At the very least you will be damp and sticky when you wake, and very often the sweat is so heavy that you need to change the sheets before you can get back into bed.

These night sweats can be ferocious. I have gone through them for long periods, waking up two or three times every night with the sweat running off me. After drying off and changing the bed, I would fall asleep quickly, only to wake up an hour later wringing wet again. The whole thing was physically exhausting and emotional demoralizing.

After one particularly awful day, when I did not have the energy to go and get myself any food or drink, I fell into bed early and went into the usual sequence of night sweats. After the first one I bounced back into bed, anxious for sleep and lay there wide awake. This was confusing because I normally fell straight back to sleep as soon as I was cool and dry. Then my temperature started to go up. Soon my mind was affected by the fever and I grew increasingly hazy and delirious as my temperature climbed. I laid there for what seemed like a month, growing hotter and hotter. Then I realized that I was not sweating, and everything fell into place. I was dehydrated, and without the sweat evaporating to cool me there was no way to control my temperature. I forced myself out of bed for a glass of water, and minutes after drinking it I was sweating again and cooling off rapidly.

This provided a valuable lesson. If you experience fevers and night sweats, make sure that you increase your intake of liquids to compensate for all the water lost through sweating. To dehydrate in a fever is dangerous and can damage you permanently. Also, every time you sweat heavily you are losing salt and other important nutrients from the body, so it is probably wise to make sure that your diet is more than adequate during these periods.

Pain-killers in small amounts are very useful to break the fever and bring your temperature down. When I was going through a bad period and expected a disturbed night, I took half or a quarter of a tablet before bedtime to help me get a good night's rest. Then, when an unexpected fever woke me up, I took the same dose and it prevented further disturbances.

SLEEP PATTERNS AND DISTURBANCES

Night sweats and fevers, as described above, are the most noticeable of the sleep disturbances that occur with this disease. The others are much less worrisome, but can still be a little disturbing. For those of us, like myself, who rarely remember their dreams, the Panavision, Technicolor epics that the illness sometimes produces can be quite shocking. Waking up with your head ringing to the sights and sounds of this unexpected dreamscape can be alarming at first.

Learn to relax and enjoy this built-in entertainment system. Think of it as a compensation for all of the difficult times.

Apart from sweats and dreams, you could find yourself waking up in the middle of the night for any number of reasons—for a drink or a snack or to go to the toilet. Then there are times when there is no good reason to wake up; you simply do. Whether or not you're hungry or thirsty, you'll often find that some food or a hot drink will send you back to sleep quickly and safely. Avoid sleeping pills, unless there really is no other option.

Disturbances of your sleep patterns are always unpleasant. When they are frequent it's like living with permanent jet lag. Every body has its own rhythms, its own preferences for when to sleep and when to wake. Many sufferers find that their illness throws their sleep patterns into total disarray, and they have to adjust their lifestyles continually to cope with irregular sleep needs.

Most of us find that we require more sleep than normal, but instead of taking it in one single block at night, our bodies tell us to rest at various points during the day. As I have already said, I have a daily "low" between four and six p.m. At that time I feel tired and drained and would like nothing better than to lie down. When I was really ill I had to sleep then. If I had deliberately kept myself awake (if that were possible), it would have weakened me and perhaps triggered a relapse. During the intense periods of illness you need all the sleep you can get, to allow your mind and body to replenish themselves. Once you achieve a convalescent state, or even remission, you can retrain your mind and body to sleep once in every 24 hours.

Make up your mind to accept the fact that while you are ill you will feel the need to sleep at odd times of the day. As long as this does not interfere too much with your sleep at night, give in to it. As you start to get better you can rest instead of sleep during the day, and this will gradually alter your sleep pattern to a more appropriate rhythm.

SWEATS

Some patients have the unpleasant experience of sweats that seem unconnected with temperature changes. These sweats can happen at any time, but are usually daytime events. The sweats are unusual in that only one part of the body might be involved. For example, the thighs, lower legs, arms, armpits, neck and back can all be affected individually. No anti-perspirant will prevent these sweats, and no deodorant can mask the odor, which is sometimes awful.

Feeling just one part of your body sweating is a very peculiar sensation, and as yet no one knows how or why these localized sweats happen. However, there is reason to believe that they are healthy. Any sweat contains wastes and toxins that the body wants to throw off. Heavy or badly smelling sweats are likely to be a simple defense mechanism that allows the body to free itself of all sorts of rubbish that has accumulated in your system. Unfortunately, it is these wastes that produce the awful smell, which can be extremely embarrassing. Console yourself with the fact that your body is protecting itself by sweating out wastes, and use the treatment described under hydrotherapy to alleviate this irritating symptom. By regularly using a therapy that causes you to sweat you can prevent both these localized sweats and the more wearing night sweats.

SECONDARY INFECTIONS

CFS is a relentless attack on your body's natural defenses. Over a period of time, your defenses become worn down to the point where you are more susceptible to other infections than you would normally be. Your immune system, which normally fights off invading germs, becomes depressed and can no longer react as quickly or effectively as it should. This allows other infections, called secondary infections, to take hold. Once established they can be very difficult to get rid of.

Some people experience this immune depression as a tendency to catch colds, flu and other bugs more often, and find that once caught they can last for weeks at a time. Others persistently get infections in the same places. My throat was a definite weak spot, and I also suffered from urethritis regularly.

Usually the secondary infections are minor. A healthy person could overcome them within a few days. However, because of the depressed state of your immune system, minor infections can become a major problem.

To take the common cold as an example, a healthy person usually overcomes the virus within a week. For a CFS patient it could take three or four weeks. And the story does not end there. Any secondary infection may stress your system beyond its ability to cope, and all your CFS symptoms may return or intensify with great speed and force.

The only truly effective way to treat secondary infections is not to get them in the first place. Prevention is certainly better and easier than cure. You may not be able to defend yourself completely against all of the many different bugs that people are prone to, but you can at least take elementary precautions. Don't visit friends and relatives who have coughs, colds, flu or any other communicable disease, and don't allow these people to visit you.

If one part of your body is particularly susceptible to infections, protect it from stress. For instance, with my throat always poised on the brink of infection, I quickly learned to cut out all the things that might irritate it. I eliminated alcohol and other strong drinks from my diet, along with hot and spicy foods. Then, the unkindest cut of all, I had to cut out as much talking as possible. These measures allowed my throat to recuperate and gave it a better chance of fighting off any new potential infections. This, in turn, helped my general health. With no recurrent throat problems, my system was that much more efficient fighting off the primary infection—CFS.

CANDIDA AND THRUSH

A yeast-like fungal microorganism known as *Candida albicans* lives quite naturally and, under normal circumstances, harmlessly in certain regions of the intestinal tract. It is only when the internal "climate" of the body changes, allowing *Candida* to breed freely, that it causes problems in the gut, with associated infections such as thrush. Among the things that are known to provoke *Candida* overgrowth are an excess of sugar in the diet, overuse of antibiotics, and the contraceptive pill.

The result of *Candida* overgrowth in the gut is a depletion of the body's natural immune response system, which in turn leads to a number of symptoms, including fatigue. It is a predisposing factor in CFS, and many patients have *Candida* problems with the related conditions of developing allergies, chronic diarrhea or constipation, oral or vaginal thrush, and other symptoms.

The drug Nystatin, an anti-fungal agent, has proved useful in controlling *Candida* overgrowth, but it is not the complete answer, and the necessary strategy is one that helps the body back to health so that the gut yeasts can be held in check naturally. Eliminate as much sugar as possible from your diet and avoid yeast-containing foods.

Another excellent treatment for *Candida* problems, and one that is entirely natural, is a regular dose of bacteria called acidophilus. You can buy it in most health food stores in capsule form and, like *Candida*, it is a normal inhabitant of our internal world. In healthy people *Candida* and acidophilus compete within the digestive tract, and this helps to keep *Candida* from getting out of control.

If you purchased acidophilus in tablet form, take them the last thing at night, and chew them thoroughly before swallowing. They taste fairly pleasant, so this is no real hardship. They can be an effective treatment for all *Candida* problems, and a preventative measure thereafter.

ALLERGIES

We all have mild allergies to something in the environment, and when we are well we can easily overlook them. If your body is weakened by illness, though, it can no longer deal with these allergies and they can come out with some force. In fact, they are a major problem for longterm patients.

Clearly you need to identify and avoid the foods you've developed allergic reactions to, but if you have severe problems see your doctor, or seek the advice of a qualified clinical ecologist.

DIGESTIVE DISORDERS

There is such a huge variety of digestive disorders that it is pointless to try to describe them all. However, one should definitely be noted: constipation. This is a common symptom that, for some reason, can complicate all the other symptoms enormously. Even when the constipation is mild it can, quite literally, make all your other symptoms feel ten times worse than they really are. Therefore, regular bowel movements are of prime importance. Obviously, it is best to prevent difficulties from arising by including lots of fiber in your diet. If you have problems, it's probably best to treat yourself with a gentle natural laxative and make as many diet improvements as you can.

DEBILITATION

In the dictionary debilitation is defined as "feebleness," and that is exactly how it feels. I doubt whether this is a distinct symptom of CFS. It is more likely that a combination of other symptoms—coldness, tiredness, weakness, lack of concentration, etc.—produces the feeling of being absolutely feeble. The best way to describe this state is that those in it have a total lack of stamina, mental and physical. If you think that debilitation describes your situation accurately, try to pinpoint the symptoms that are active in your case, and treat them instead of the overall feebleness. Treating the precise problem will produce the best results.

MISCELLANEOUS

There is a group of symptoms that are not in themselves major problems, but that can produce difficulties and worry if you're not prepared for them. Very often these symptoms can be the first to appear, acting as an early warning system and alerting you to the fact that you need to take care of yourself or relapse into another bout of illness.

Pallor

Pallor is one classic early warning sign. "Pallor" simply means "paleness" and it is recognized medically as a sign of the illness. In practical terms it means that you go white. This can happen at any time up to several hours before the beginning of an attack or the worsening of symptoms. It also happens when you get overtired or are in danger of exhaustion. It is an infallible indicator of your state of health and should always be taken as a warning. Unfortunately, the patient is rarely aware of this paleness and has to rely on other people to point it out.

CFS Throat

CFS throat is not, as far as I know, recognized medically, but you should learn to look out for it. It is a slightly gruff quality in the voice, caused by a thickening of your saliva. It seems like a mild cold—your throat feels a little bit clogged up. If you don't clear your throat regularly your voice tends to be rough and unreliable. Your saliva becomes noticeably thicker than usual and may get creamy in texture and taste.

This is particularly obvious after a drink of cold water. This throat condition can last for days, weeks or months at a time, and always indicates that you are in a weakened state.

Nausea

Nausea is another good warning sign for those who suffer from it. Nauseous attacks at night or early in the morning, sometimes leading to vomiting, often foreshadow an increase in problems. The other pattern of nausea—attacks lasting only minutes at any time of day—is not such a reliable indicator, since these attacks may happen during any period of the illness.

Urine Retention Problems

Problems of urine retention tend to happen towards the end of a bout of illness. Having to go to the toilet frequently (and when you have to go, you *really* have to go), can be embarrassing and awkward. However, it is a good indicator of your convalescence. As long as the symptom persists, remember that you should be taking things relatively easy.

Appetite Disorders

Appetite disorders come in various forms at different times during the illness. During the worst of the bouts, you may find that the sight or even the thought of food is enough to make you sick. Alternatively, you could be permanently ravenous. If you were turned off by food during the illness, you will probably find that in convalescence you will have sudden, sharp pangs of hunger. Within minutes you can go from being comfortably full to feeling as though you had been months without food. The sensation can amount almost to panic. Always give in to these hungers and get some food into your body as soon as possible. Otherwise, your strength may drain away quickly, leaving you feeling weak and ill. Many people carry around some biscuits, an apple or a chocolate bar, just in case one of these starvation attacks occurs. This is a very sensible idea.

Photophobia & Sound Sensitivity

Photophobia is the technical term for light sensitivity, which is a very common problem with CFS patients. Sound sensitivity is also common. Both symptoms are associated with migraine-type headaches, but they may also be experienced separately. In these conditions bright light or loud sounds may cause pain in the eyes and head, or ears and head respectively. Some people, like myself, find that they have no problems with artificial light but that sunlight is painful. Others find that direct light of any sort causes no difficulty, but sunlight through a window is unbearable. There is very little you can do about these conditions, but as your health improves they will gradually disappear. Meanwhile, you might invest in a pair of sunglasses or some earplugs, if your environment is a noisy one.

Swollen Glands

Many people find that their glands are another infallible sign that a bout of illness is approaching. The glands may be those in your throat but those in the armpits or groin may also react. When these glands become hard, swollen or painful, you are being told in no uncertain terms to take care of yourself—as your system is weakened. Incidentally, it is because of this condition that CFS is so often wrongly diagnosed as glandular fever.

THE MENTAL AND EMOTIONAL SYMPTOMS

Having examined the physical problems of CFS, let's take a look at the other end of the spectrum—the mental and emotional symptoms. We know so little about how the mind works that any description of that process in health or illness, can only be approximate. Take the following symptoms as signposts only. Your mental and emotional experience of CFS will be like your mind—totally unique.

DEPRESSION

Usually we use the word "depression" to cover a mixture of feelings, such as boredom, frustration, lack of motivation and general lack of fulfillment. This is an adequate definition in day-to-day life, but real depression is something else again: You feel that you cannot help yourself, cannot make a constructive move and cannot expect things to improve. In this state you believe, beyond a shadow of a doubt, that things can only get worse. You feel trapped in a web of circumstance that you cannot escape. There seems to be no hope, except that oblivion will release you from the torment of living. This true depression is a crippling illness.

CFS causes depression by affecting the part of the brain that helps to control our emotional states. The degree of depression varies from person to person and from day to day, but even the happiest of people can find themselves in despair. Many patients may tell you of their suicidal thoughts and feelings. Because depression often strikes when physical symptoms are at their worst, the world including your own body can indeed seem a hopeless, helpless, loveless place.

The depression can drop over you within minutes, like a cloud moving over the sun. Happily, it can lift just as quickly and unexpectedly, leaving you feeling as if you have been hit by an invisible truck and miraculously escaped unhurt.

The key to dealing with all depressions, whether of the everyday or the despairing variety, is to keep one fact in mind: You will get over it. Commonsense and past experience tell you that within a day or a week or a month, you will be looking back at the down time and wondering what it was all about. If you can maintain even the slightest optimism and belief in yourself, you will win through more quickly.

Most states of depression you encounter with CFS can be overcome fairly easily. However, if you find yourself in a very low state, and it continues beyond your ability to cope, don't hesitate to seek help from your doctor. Anti-depressant drugs may be a sensible treatment for this phase of your illness. By this I don't mean tranquilizers. Unlike tranquilizers, anti-depressants need to be taken daily for a number of weeks before they become effective in relieving symptoms. In some cases they can literally be a "life saver," but take great care because it is easy to overdose; there are side effects; and you can become addicted.

If you are at all unsure about whether a prescribed drug is helping you, go straight back to your doctor. Finally, make up your mind to use anti-depressants as little as possible, not just to lessen the chance of side effects and addiction, but also because it is much healthier for you to rely on your own ability to beat the illness rather than on drugs. Using anti-depressants is not a bad thing when you need them, but it is best to use the relief they provide to find a less harmful therapy that will help you to maintain your optimism.

MEMORY

Almost everyone I have spoken to has mentioned memory lapses as one of the most frustrating aspects of this illness. During bouts of illness, this amnesia can become extensive. Hardly any information is retained in either the short-term or the long-term memory, so making notes has to become a way of life. During convalescent periods, memory returns to a certain extent, but there may still be lapses. Names, faces, telephone numbers and all sorts of other information disappear from your mind completely or become so vague and misty that your memory cannot be trusted. Coping with this can be embarrassing and amusing by turns. Forgetting to buy an important present or to make an important phone call can be extremely unfortunate—and not only for yourself. On the other hand, forgetting your old friends' names can easily be turned into a joke if they understand your situation. People are usually very understanding about such things and are prepared to join in the fun if you treat the problem lightheartedly.

I well remember a three-way conversation I had with two other patients, Sue and Les. We all knew each other's names well, but kept having trouble. On pain of death I could not recall their proper names, but persisted in calling them Laura and Mike. Les forgot Sue's name totally, and called me Paul. Sue called me Mike, but remembered Les accurately. What was supposed to be a serious interview become quietly hysterical and we ended up giving each other rounds of applause whenever we hit the right name.

It really won't help to try to force your memory into cooperating. The stress will simply aggravate your illness and cause more lapses than ever. As the illness recedes, our memories return to something approaching normality. In the meantime, it's a good idea to learn to make notes of the important things and laugh off the rest.

COMPREHENSION

Comprehension is the ability to understand the things you see or hear—the ability to make sense of information. With CFS the simplest things became quite beyond my understanding. Once, during a medical examination, a doctor asked me to stand up. I did not have the foggiest idea what that meant. It was just a meaningless noise. When understanding finally dawned, I felt humiliated at my own stupidity.

This lack of comprehension can be devastating, encompassing sight, sound, touch, taste and smell. In extreme cases the person can barely understand anything and lives as if isolated from the rest of the world.

Usually the problem does not get as severe, but it does present difficulties to most patients: Books, TV, magazines and even conversation can become quite pointless because they are totally confusing. There is little that will dramatically improve this specific problem except improving your general health, but several therapies such as autogenics, Bach flower remedies, and royal jelly can help.

In convalescence you may find the lack of comprehension continuing in its mild forms, getting noticeably worse when you are tired. I found that the things I heard were first to regain their meaning, followed slowly and incompletely by visual comprehension. Even now, I still have difficulty with the written word. My spelling used to be excellent, but now I am mildly dyslexic. I cannot recognize a word when it is spelled incorrectly without a massive exertion of will. No doubt the manuscript of this book was full of mistakes—my thanks to the editor who must have worked hard to clean it up for publication.

Concentration, or rather the lack of it, also deserves a mention here. Many people find that their ability to focus their minds is badly impaired by CFS. During the worst stages of the illness it becomes difficult to concentrate on anything for more than a few minutes—or even seconds— at a time. Personally, I have no doubt that forcing my mind to concentrate was harmful during these periods. The effort of concentration needed to make an important phone call or answer a letter left me very weak and ill. It seems there was little difference between body and mind in this respect. When I pushed my body beyond the limits of its strength, I suffered for it in the following days. The same was true of my mind. In convalescence I needed to push my body a little further each day to build up my strength, always being sure not to overextend myself. Again, the same was true of my mind. Gradually I exercised my mental muscles in the same way that I exercised my physical ones. Little by little the strength returned to both.

COORDINATION AND BALANCE

Lack of coordination is one of the more trying symptoms, because it can appear to be dreadful clumsiness. One woman who was severely affected described herself as "a mobile accident zone."

The appearance of clumsiness is caused by the fact that the patients are no longer fully aware of exactly where their hands and feet are. Most people can reach for a cup, for example, and know almost by instinct when their hand is in the right position to pick it up safely. When your coordination is impaired, this instinct can lead you astray. You feel as though your hand is safely positioned, but in fact it can be inches away from the object you are trying to grasp. The result of this is an endless succession of dropped or knocked over cups, plates, vases, trays and anything else that comes to hand—or foot (trips, stumbles and falls).

Coordination problems are often accompanied by, and aggravated by, a lack of balance. Sometimes this takes the form of dizziness or vertigo, but more often it is simply an inability to stand or move straight. Walking down a perfectly ordinary corridor, I used to reel from wall to wall as though the floor beneath my feet were a wildly tossing ship. Getting into the right position to enter a door without damaging it or myself became quite a problem! It occurred to me that the doctors had overlooked one obvious symptom of CFS—bruised shoulders from continual impact with walls and door frames.

If you have difficulty with coordination or balance, you need to take things more carefully. Realize that your body is temporarily unable to be accurate in positioning itself, and compensate by taking a little more time and effort as you move. This may not save some of your favorite pottery from grief, but it should reduce the wear and tear on your shoulders.

EMOTIONAL PROBLEMS

There are two problems that can be as difficult for your friends and family as they are for you. The first one is mood swings.

Mood Swings

Mood swings affect everybody all of the time. Many of us go through life feeling up one minute and down the next. Very often these changes can be triggered by seemingly unimportant things, but the effects color our outlook for as long as the mood lasts. With CFS patients, mood swings can be very violent and very fast—euphoric highs followed within minutes by plummeting lows.

In the high state you feel on top of the world, happy and carefree. You give off a glow of good humor and laugh at anything or nothing at all. In the low state tears take over and the carefree feeling turns into despondency.

Even in far milder forms these sudden changes can confuse and frighten the people around you. The best thing you can do is to tell them exactly what is going on inside you. Once they understand that your mood swings are not their fault, they can stop worrying and start to help. This also relieves you of the guilt you may feel for exposing your friends and family to such emotional turmoil.

Anti-Social Behavior

The second emotional problem is a tendency to go through anti-social phases. It can be distressing to have good friends come to see you, and no sooner have they arrived than you cannot wait to see them go. The problem is even greater if it is members of your own household that you cannot bear to have around.

The reason for these anti-social periods is not yet known. Obviously, at least part of it is that you're feeling weak and tired and are perhaps confused and in pain. It's natural at these times to want to seclude yourself. However, the irregular suddenness and intensity of these feelings leads me to think that they are a true by-product, a true symptom, of the illness.

Whatever the cause of these feelings, the cure is simple. Talk about them. Take the trouble to explain to your nearest and dearest that you are going through periods when you just have to be on your own. Once they understand that this is no reflection on your relationship with them, but simply a part of your illness, they will be happy to let you have solitude when you need it and welcome you back when you are ready to communicate again.

This, then, is our list of symptoms. Let me stress again that just because they are on the list doesn't mean that every person who catches CFS will suffer from them. Nobody will suffer from all of them. You will probably find that a few will be with you fairly frequently; others may come and go and some may not affect you at all. Having read the list, you have been forewarned and forearmed. You need not spend precious time and energy worrying about what is happening to your body. You can, instead, focus all your attention on combating your symptoms with all the available therapies.

4

THE TREATMENT

When they consider moving away from orthodox medical care into alternative medicine, people often ask, "Will it work for me?" Unfortunately, this question cannot be answered with a simple "Yes" or "No." The only real answer is "Yes, if you find the right therapy." This may lead you to believe that alternative therapies are erratic and that their results will vary from person to person. This is true, but exactly the same must be said for traditional treatments. The drugs a doctor prescribes will work for one person but not for another. The fact that they often work well is a testament to the skill of the doctor in choosing the right treatment for the right patient. An equally skilled alternative therapist will have the same degree of success.

It is foolish to fall into the trap of thinking only in terms of one type of medicine. Orthodox and alternative therapies are not mutually exclusive. They can work happily together, each bringing about benefits to the patient. Remember, however, to keep all you caregivers informed of your treatments. If your homeopath, for example, puts you on a course of pills at the same time that your doctor does, make sure that each one knows what the other has prescribed. There is little chance of the two treatments reacting badly together, but orthodox drugs may sometimes inhibit the action of natural treatments and vice versa.

Alternative therapies spring from an entirely different outlook on health from orthodox medicine. Traditional medical practitioners tend to think of the body as a machine, and they treat the parts of the machine that are not working smoothly. In this sense, they treat the disease and not the patient. Alternative practitioners like to think of the patient as a whole unit (hence the term "holistic medicine") composed of mind and body. They believe that both aspects of self must be treated to cure any problem. They often consider illness the outward physical reflection of an internal (mental, emotional or spiritual) problem. Therefore they work to cure the ailment by treating the problem at its roots in the patient's inner self. Bear this attitude in mind when you are considering alternative therapies and they may not seem quite so illogical or "other worldly."

Another noticeable difference between orthodox medicine and alternative medicine is the speed at which the treatments work. We are all conditioned to the fact that tablets from the doctor work very speedily usually within days if not hours. Natural preparations usually work much more slowly, gently easing their way into your system and correcting imbalances. Of course, speedy cures can and do occur with natural remedies, but be prepared for the fact that you may have to be a patient and allow extra time for this natural magic to work.

All of the therapies listed here have been tried by me or by other CFS patients and have proven effective against certain symptoms. Don't be afraid to try different therapies—or different combinations of them—from those listed here. Follow your own instincts and intuitions faithfully, and try what seems right to you.

Finding an effective treatment depends largely on how vigorously you pursue it. No one, as yet, has discovered a treatment that is effective for most patients most of the time. Therefore, it is up to you to seek out those things that will provide a measure of relief from your particular combination of symptoms. Some of the therapies mentioned in this book may work only partially for you, giving you only a temporary respite. If that happens, don't be dismayed. Temporary relief is far better than none at all, and use this period to explore other treatments. The next one you try might be the one that does the trick.

When you find a therapy that works, stick with it. There's no point in abandoning a successful treatment to try another that might be better, but alternatively might fail. Instead add another therapy, which will work hand-in-hand with your successful one, to your routine. In this way you will gradually build up a network of interlocking treatments that together will alleviate all your symptoms. Eventually you will reach a point where you are in remission, and only need to use the therapies often enough to maintain your state of health. At this point it would be wise to use them occasionally as a purely preventive measure, to keep you on the straight and narrow path of health.

For a beginner, the world of alternative medicine can seem a strange and complex place. The majority of us were brought up to consider Western medicine the norm. With a little knowledge and effort we can understand why a doctor prescribes a particular drug for a particular illness, because the whole system is based on sound logical principles. Alternative therapies often seem to be based on ways of thought that are different—sometimes even ridiculous. However, each system of thought is perfectly logical and perfectly sensible within its own context. It is only when you compare them with each other that they seem strange.

The system of thought underlying Western medicine is

that most ill-health is caused by external influences, such as germs, lack of proper nutrition and so forth. Because we have been taught this since childhood, we tend to accept it without question. The philosophy underlying many of the therapies in this book is that most ill-health is caused by internal influences—mental, emotional or spiritual problems that push the body out of its natural healthy balance. At first glance this new idea seems very odd. How can an internal problem cause you to catch flu, or, for that matter, CFS? It seems much more logical to assume that environmental influences are responsible for disease. But this theory of external cause has a major stumbling block. With every breath of air and every bite of food we put germs into our bodies—that is a fact of life. Why do some of these germs affect us and some not? How can we go through weeks of winter surrounded by germs of all types without catching anything? And having escaped illness for weeks, why do we suddenly come down with a cold? Something within us must have changed, preventing our bodies from destroying the germs efficiently. It is reasonable to believe that this internal change emanates from the mental, emotional or even spiritual levels of our beings.

There are, no doubt, grains of truth underlying all of the therapies mentioned in this book. They each have something unique to offer. If they also seem to have something ridiculous within them, we should be very wary of throwing stones. Western medicine is a glass house built on a supremely ridiculous fact: We only go to doctors when we are ill. To the Chinese—and some other peoples with systems of medicine far more ancient than our own—this is patently absurd. To them, a doctor is responsible for keeping his patients *healthy*, not for curing them when they are ill. He sees them when they are well and makes every effort to keep them that way. If one of his patients should fall ill, the doctor's reputation suffers badly and he receives no payment for the duration of the illness. What could be more sensible, more logical or more practical than this? Prevention is absolutely the best way of treating any disease known to man.

As you start to explore alternative therapies you will find yourself encountering many philosophies. If you study them a little, you will soon have your concepts of health and illness turned upside down. As your horizons expand, these new ideas can give a whole new meaning to life. Of course, it is not necessary to know anything at all about the theory behind a therapy to make it work for you. Even if you have no interest in the ideas behind each system of thought, the therapies will be enormously helpful.

When trying the therapies, start with those that have the best chance of relieving your worst symptoms. If you haven't alleviated the problem within a month or so, try another type of treatment. As soon as you have some success, start working on your lesser problems in the same way. When the minor symptoms improve, try new treatments, always starting with those that have proved successful in the past. If healing, for example, helped you overcome your tiredness, then in all probability it will help you with nausea and coldness as well. Keep exploring and you will eventually overcome your illness.

THE THERAPIES

ACUPUNCTURE AND ACUPRESSURE

Acupuncture and acupressure were two of the first therapies from oriental medicine to establish themselves in the West. They are now popular enough to be available in all major cities and in many smaller towns too.

The most important writings on acupuncture are a collection of 34 books known as the *Nei Ching*. This collection took over 1,500 years to complete, with the final chapter being written about 3,000 years ago. The acupuncture techniques described in these books were carried out with "stone piercers" or "stone borers," but by Neolithic times the Chinese were using needles of bone or bamboo. The discovery of metal marked a major development in the science of acupuncture; iron, silver and many alloys have been used to make needles. Today, the acupuncturist uses needles of processed stainless steel.

Originally, it was thought that the substance the needles were made from cured disease, but later it was established that it was the method of application that produced the beneficial effects. Certain points on the skin affected and perhaps controlled the working of certain organs of the body. Using needles on these points affected the associated organs, which could be healed of disease by this method.

Underlying acupuncture and acupressure is the theory that two flows of energy, called *yin* and *yang*, exist in the body. These are contained within an overall conception of energy known as the life force of *Ch'i*. These energies are part of everything we do, think or feel. When they flow freely, and are in balance with each other, they produce what we know as health. When the flow is blocked or unbalanced, disease results. The Chinese discovered that this vital energy circulates through the body in the same way as blood. The channels it flows in are called meridians.

There are 26 major meridians, each associated with an organ or body function. Acupuncture/acupressure points occur where the meridians emerge at the surface of the body. There are more than 800 of these points, and new ones are being discovered continually. By piercing the skin (acupuncture) or massaging it (acupressure) at these points, the therapist stimulates or sedates the energy flow. This restores the energy balance within the body, bringing about a functioning equilibrium.

Every single point produces a different effect on our energy and thus in our bodies. Learning about each point and its effect is a lifetime's study. For this reason, the practice of acupuncture is a very complex business and best left to the professionals. Acupressure is much safer to use on yourself, and there are many books on the market that will introduce you to the major pressure points and tell you how to stimulate them correctly.

The main benefits that can come to a CFS patient from acupuncture or acupressure treatments are pain relief and increased vitality and strength. Individuals for whom it works well also report various minor benefits including improvements in vision and comprehension. I can offer no personal tips about this because I have always been unresponsive to these therapies. I have occasionally found acupressure useful for stress relief, but I have never experienced any major benefit from either treatment—which puts me in a small minority.

Acupuncture

However, I do have enough experience to answer the most common questions about acupuncture. "Do the needles hurt?" is a frequent one, and the answer is "No." Very often you will be entirely unaware that the needle has been inserted until you look. The next question is often, "What do you feel?" The answer depends on how sensitive you are to the subtle energies of your own body. If you are very sensitive, you may feel a range of responses—warmth, coolness, tingling or a general sensation of what might be called release. The sensations are usually quite pleasant.

In these AIDS-aware days, many people are turning away from acupuncture because of the possibility of catching the HIV virus. Their fear is entirely groundless. No reputable practitioner would ever use unsterilized needles, and very often the needles will be sterilized in your presence. Feel free to check this with your practitioners. They will fully understand your worries and do everything possible to reassure you.

Acupressure

As far as acupressure is concerned, I can vouch for its effectiveness even though it does not help me personally. I learned the basics of the technique to use with massage, and over the years many of my friends have benefited from my use of it. It is very simple and usually immediately effective, though it can be briefly painful. This is because instead of a fine needle you are using your finger or thumb to put pressure on a point. Therefore, you are pressing and massaging the entire surrounding area too. If deep massage is required to stimulate the pressure point fully, you may be uncomfortable for a brief period.

Finding out whether this therapy is right for you is fairly quick and simple. If it is going to be helpful, the benefits generally are obvious very rapidly—sometimes immediately after the first session. If, after three or four sessions, you are still feeling no better, then it may be wise to try other forms of treatment. Acupuncture and acupressure, like the other therapies, are completely safe in various combinations, but they are particularly harmonious with reflexology and healing.

AUTOGENIC TRAINING

Developed by J. H. Schultz in the early part of this century, autogenic training is a unique combination of hypnotic and relaxation techniques. It is often used by sufferers of long-term or chronic sickness, because in the later stages of the therapy the individual can devise exercises that affect those specific areas of the mind and body that are giving them trouble. In effect, the therapy is tailored to the precise needs of each individual.

The therapy started almost by accident when some students of Schultz, who were studying autohypnosis (see page 84), started entering a strange mental state during their practice periods. The state was one of deep physical and mental relaxation and mental clarity. The students reported that after a few minutes of this they emerged refreshed and invigorated, with all fatigue and tension gone. This prompted Schultz to start experimenting to find out more about the recuperative powers of this state of mind.

His experiments were very successful. The most important discovery, which led directly to the development of autogenic training, was that if the subject concentrated on a positive thought while in this state, improvements in mental and physical well-being came about according to the directions contained in the positive thought. In this way people could gain control of their own energies in a way that had not been known before.

By the 1920s, Schultz had evolved and simplified the technique to create a range of standard exercises to bring harmony to all aspects of mind and body. These are called the Autogenic Standard Series, and they form the central core of the therapy. Each exercise involves concentrating passively on a series of mental commands while lying with eyes closed in a quiet room. The exercises have to be practiced several times a day, until you can voluntarily shift from a state of high mental or physical energy to a lower one.

The major drawback to this therapy is the time it takes to master the basic exercises. A person who is healthy in mind and body may take several months to learn the processes fully, and a person who is physically or mentally depleted may find that the learning period has to be extended considerably. Unfortunately, it is only when you have mastered the basics that you can develop the mental commands tailored to your own situation or illness.

Even with this drawback, I would still recommend autogenic training. It is a simple, safe and effective way to make sure that your mental and physical energies remain relatively free and healthy. What's more, it also makes you realize that you and you alone are responsible for your state of body and mind—a fact that we all tend to overlook.

Obviously, the positive mental commands you concentrate on during the exercises do help, but in the case of CFS the deep relaxation alone is enough to bring about benefits. Almost everyone who tries a therapy that includes some relaxation work is surprised by the benefits it brings. I suspect that most people think, "When you are constantly tired and weak, who needs to be relaxed?" The truth is that relaxation refreshes your mind and body in a way that nothing else does. People who learn autogenics, autohypnosis or any other form of deep relaxation soon realize that a few minutes of proper relaxing is more refreshing than hours of sleep. In this sense, at least, autogenics can be greatly helpful.

The major benefits of this therapy are the refreshing of physical energy and the renewing of mental concentration and comprehension. You will notice improvements in these areas even when you're just studying the technique. You may also be able to control other major symptoms, such as muscular pain, but this ability varies from person to person. Once you master the technique, you can use it to reduce or eliminate many minor symptoms. Altogether, it is a very effective therapy if you have the time, energy and will to study it fully.

Autogenics instructors are sometimes difficult to locate, but it is possible to teach yourself the basics of the technique from books. Autogenic exercises are completely compatible with all other therapies.

AROMATHERAPY

This therapy is one of the most elegant and pleasurable I have ever studied. It is also one of the most consistently successful.

Aromatherapy, as the name suggests, relies on the aroma of natural substances to produce its therapeutic effects. The origin of the fragrances can be herbs, woods, spices, flowers or resins, but in every case only the pure oil that gives the substance its natural fragrance is used. This oil, once distilled, is the essence of the plant or resin it came from, so it is often sold as essential oil as well as aromatherapy oil.

Every practitioner and student of this ancient craft seems to have his or her own suggestions as to why fragrances should have a medicinal effect. Some reason that using these plant essences is akin to herbalism. Some claim that the natural fragrances affect the unconscious mind and thus heal the body. I have met more than one person who believes that the oil captures the spirit of the plant in it its essence, and it is this that heals the user. Whatever the reason for its success, it works well for almost everyone who tries it.

The simplicity of this therapy is its greatest virtue. You can use it at any time and under any circumstances whatsoever. The simplest method is to dab a little of the appropriate oil on the inside of your nostrils, so that you are continually inhaling the fragrance. Alternatively, you can place a drop on a radiator, candle or light bulb (before switching it on), which will fill the room with a therapeutic aroma. Adding essential oil to a basic massage oil brings a new dimension to both therapies, and scenting your bath water with a few drops of pure essence produces immediate benefits to mind and body.

Selecting the appropriate oil to counteract your symptoms can be confusing for the beginner. There are dozens of oils, each with a different therapeutic value, and you can combine them to develop literally thousands of new scents. Don't worry about trying to mix them at first. Stick to using single oils until you have found the ones that work for you; then start combining them in equal proportions. Test these simple mixtures and adjust the proportions according to your own findings. In no time at all you will be confidently mixing all sorts of fragrant brews for yourself, friends and family.

To help you take your first steps in this productive and entertaining therapy, I have prepared a list of oils that many CFS sufferers find beneficial. Select your first oils from this list, and then add other oils recommended to help with your particular problems. Any aromatherapy book will be helpful in this respect.

Oil of Lavender

Tiredness, weakness, pain and coldness all produce tension, so the first oil you should think about trying is Oil of Lavender, which is a strong relaxant. As we've seen, relaxation is extremely important because it allows the mind and body to release tensions and toxins and draw in new energy. The light and flowery fragrance of lavender is soothing, melting away both physical and mental fatigue. After a bad day, a few drops of this essence in a warm bath prepares you for a night of good, refreshing sleep. Another benefit of lavender is its versatility. You can mix it with almost any other oil with pleasing results.

Oil of Lemon

Oil of Lemon (not Oil of Lemongrass) is one that people tend to shy away from, imagining that it will have a bitter, acidic scent. In fact, it is very pleasant, with a fresh, cool fragrance that produces a calming effect on the mind. Its primary use is to unwind and refresh the mind, though it also helps to prevent night sweats and fevers. If you mix lemon and lavender, the two scents combine to produce the aromatic equivalent of knock-out drops. In periods of disturbed or unrefreshing sleep, this combination is invaluable. It helps you to sleep well and wake up feeling rested.

Oil of Peppermint

Like lemon, Oil of Peppermint is useful in the prevention of night sweats and fevers, as it has a pronounced cooling effect. However, peppermint is best used in the morning as it is an invigorating scent, an energizer for mind and body. It also regulates the whole digestive system gently but firmly. Note: use with care; it can irritate your skin.

Oil of Basil

Oil of Basil is another invigorating aroma, but in a slightly different way. It lifts the spirits and clears the mind. In a bath it produces a slightly electric tingling sensation that is pleasantly stimulating, but be wary of using more than a couple of drops at a time. In larger amounts it can irritate your skin quite painfully. Also be careful when mixing basil with other oils. It mixes well with essences drawn from other herbs or from woods, but not with some of the lighter, more flowery fragrances.

Oil of Rosemary

Oil of Rosemary is excellent against lethargy and early morning sluggishness. Its clean, sharp fragrance stimulates the mind and body, and prepares you for a new day.

Oil of Clary Sage

Oil of Clary Sage (not Oil of Sage) is another good tonic, suitable for use any time in the day. The nutty, floral scent is warming and soothing, and you will probably find that it leaves you feeling in high spirits. Another versatile oil, it can be blended with confidence.

Oil of Orange

Oil of Orange (or Oil of Sweet Orange) is a good addition to your collection because of its all-over helpfulness. It is refreshing and uplifting and helps to keep you at a mental and physical peak.

Oil of Geranium

Oil of Geranium is a remarkable cleanser of both body and mind, and I highly recommend it for those days when you feel slow and unresponsive, as though your system were clogged up. Another benefit of geranium (also called Rose Geranium) is its effectiveness in harmonizing troubled emotions, so it is useful to keep handy as an antidote to the whole range of emotional problems that can accompany CFS.

Using the Oils

Most of the oils you can buy are completely safe to use, though of course none should be taken internally except under professional supervision. However, a few oils, such as peppermint and basil, may irritate your skin. If you plan to apply the oils directly to your skin, as in a massage, then it is safest to dilute them beforehand. All of the oils can be diluted with any vegetable oil without losing their therapeutic effect. You can purchase specially blended base oils to dilute them with, but for the ultimate in luxurious skin care, I would suggest that you dilute the essences with Oil of Sweet Almond (Almond Oil), which is extremely beneficial to the skin and available inexpensively at health food stores.

Although most of these oils are widely available through health shops, department stores and other retail outlets, they are quite expensive, which can be a drawback. The reason for the expense is that only tiny quantities of oil exist in each plant; so hundreds of plants must be processed to produce each bottle of pure essence. Often oils are cheaper by mail order. The classified sections of many health magazines include ads, so it shouldn't be too difficult to locate a supplier.

Some CFS patients believe there is another drawback to aromatherapy: The relief it provides is temporary and daily treatment may be necessary. To me, this is a short-sighted attitude. Nothing yet known permanently alleviates CFS, and, until we find something that does, any therapy that relieves the symptoms is worthwhile. The relief provided by aromatherapy and other treatments may be short-term, but if it allows you to think and feel positive for a while, that is a major factor in your favor on a day-to-day basis.

BACH FLOWER REMEDIES

In the year before the First World War, Dr. Edward Bach received his diploma in Public Health from Cambridge. This was just one of the many qualifications and distinctions he earned during his long and productive career in medicine. He worked in both medical practice and research, and has been credited with excellent achievements in both fields. However, it was not until his retirement that he began the work that has kept his name in the public eye ever since.

On retiring, Dr. Bach turned away from the drugs and surgery that had been his tools as a traditional physician, and began to experiment with the healing powers of plants and trees. He fully accepted the belief that nature provides everything man needs, and set about finding natural remedies for disease.

His research led him to conclusions that were far in advance of the science of his time. He stated that illness was the result of, or the "crystallization" of, negative mental attitudes. Now, with our greater understanding of mind and body and how they work together as an inseparable unit, we are just beginning to understand and agree, but half a century ago it was a revolutionary statement for a physician to make.

Having accepted the idea that disease was a psychological rather than a physical problem, Dr. Bach realized that treating the physical symptoms of any disease was not enough. To achieve a complete cure, the psychological "weakness" had to be rectified. At this point it was natural for him to turn to the plants and trees that he loved in his search for cures of the mind.

Eventually Dr. Bach evolved a whole new theory of treatment. He insisted that treating disease was incorrect and taught that the patient's inner self needed to be treated, as the cause of the illness lay there. He insisted the therapist ignore all symptoms, examining only the patient's temperament to uncover the negative mental attitude that caused the difficulty. It was this inner dis-ease that had to be treated every time.

Dr. Bach listed the major causes of negativity—fear, uncertainty, lack of optimism, etc.—and treated them with preparations made from plants and trees. His method of making these preparations was simple. He picked the appropriate flower and allowed it to stand in water for an hour in direct sunlight. He found that this process transferred some substance or energy from the flower into the water, which became sparkling and lively. The patient was advised to drink a few drops of this lively water several times a day.

The fact that this therapy has persisted in use and is becoming increasingly popular, is a testament to its effectiveness. The original 38 flower remedies isolated by Dr. Bach are still available, and they are still prepared according to his original method.

The benefits of this therapy are its simplicity and effectiveness, but it does not work for everyone. If it is successful for you, you may find that the remedies alleviate or cure all of the mental and emotional symptoms of CFS, radically improving your physical state. This physical improvement seems to come about because the therapy drastically reduces stress levels, which gives the body a chance to heal itself. The drawbacks are that the therapy is not widely available compared with, for instance, acupuncture. Also, unless you are very skillful at analyzing your own emotional states, it is wiser to go to a professional practitioner for diagnosis and treatment. You can study the subject from books if no practitioner is available, and ads in health magazines are a good way to locate suppliers.

COLONIC IRRIGATION

This rather odd therapy has had bursts of popularity over the years, but has never become established on a wide scale. It is seldom used in traditional medicine, and its claims as an alternative therapy have never, as far as I know, been substantiated. It has been suggested as a suitable treatment for CFS and that is why I'm including it here.

Colonic irrigation is a standard part of the regimen in some health spas and naturopathic clinics. Based on the same principles of hygiene and comfort as the enema, colonic irrigation requires more complicated equipment and affects a larger area of the body. The procedure is simple. For a varying period (usually 30 to 45 minutes) water at body temperature is injected into the rectum. The water flows out again via a two-way tube. Irrigation is more effective than an enema because it reaches above the normal defecation area, into the descending and transverse colon. As the water is washed in and out it detaches any old fecal matter that adheres to these areas.

Usually colonic irrigation is recommended only after two or three days of fasting, so that all feces and digestive residue have passed out of the colon. This is not the only limitation to its use. Conditions such as diverticulitis, certain types of colitis and malignant growths can be vastly aggravated by this therapy. Normally, it should also be avoided in cases of greatly reduced vitality. As CFS reduces vitality to a large degree, it is questionable as to whether this therapy is advisable for the majority of patients.

One side effect of colonic irrigation is usually considered a problem, but may be of benefit to CFS patients. During irrigation many of the normal digestive bacteria are washed out of the colon. As I have already noted, *Candida* bacteria reside in the digestive system and can cause problems for some patients when they get out of control. Washing out these masses of bacteria may be a good treatment for people who have severe problems in this area. Also, irrigation is effective in controlling constipation, which can be of great benefit, but there are simpler ways of achieving the same result.

Usually this treatment is prescribed for chronic conditions in which proper elimination of body wastes may be vitally important—catarrh, gastric troubles, skin disorders, etc. It should always be accompanied by strict dietary control.

There seems little logical reason to put colonic irrigation high on your list of appropriate therapies. Having said that, I must add that a few people have found it helpful, and throughout its long history the therapy has always had its devotees. Mae West, for example, swore by it as a necessity for health and beauty, and often practiced it daily.

If you decide to try colonic irrigation, do so only under the direct supervision of qualified medical personnel.

DIET

There is no suggestion whatsoever that diet causes or can cure CFS. However, during the illness your body may require different foods in different amounts from your normal intake. Adjusting your diet can help to prevent or remedy a worsening of your symptoms. If your body requires different foods from normal, you may experience cravings and aversions or just a general dissatisfaction with what you are eating. These feelings are your body's way of telling you of what it needs to function properly, and it is usually wise to give in to them.

Aversions

Aversions are the simplest to spot, and should always be obeyed without question. Many patients develop an aversion to alcohol, for example. And that's a good thing. Drinking even small amounts can produce an immediate worsening of all symptoms. Why this should happen is not known, but happen it does. Obviously, your metabolism is no longer in a fit state to deal with alcohol, so it is wise to cut it out altogether. Your tolerance for alcohol will gradually increase as you get better.

Tea is another common aversion. I was a regular tea drinker until I discovered that my several cups a day were worsening the illness. As I could drink decaffeinated coffee with no ill effects, I assume it was the caffeine in tea that harmed a weakened and overstressed system. I tried decaffeinated tea for a while, and found that it produced no ill effects. Unfortunately it made such a revolting brew that it was worse than drinking no tea at all.

There may be some aversions that are peculiar to yourself—foods and drinks that have a negative affect on you and you alone. These are easy to discover. Within minutes, or at most an hour, of having them you will start to feel bad. If you think that something is affecting you in this way, you can make sure by carrying out this simple test: Eat normally but avoid the suspect food for a day or two. The next morning, eat nothing for three or four hours after getting up. Then eat a normal-sized portion of the suspect food. If it is bad for you, you will feel worse almost immediately, and you can avoid that food in future.

Using this simple exclusion test I discovered that potato chips and pickled onions were extremely detrimental to my well-being. Either of these things would send my temperature rocketing and make me dizzy and nauseated. It may be that prior to my illness I had an allergy to them, but it was so mild that it never gave me any real problem. With my system weakened by illness, any allergy would become much more obvious and would be a serious strain on my defenses, complicating all the other symptoms.

Cravings

Cravings are sometimes harder to deal with because giving in to them indiscriminately can create difficulties in the long term. A frequent craving is for sugar. Sometimes your body's demands for sweet things can last for weeks at a time. If you give in to it, you may be causing any number of problems for yourself in the future. Try things like sugar-free chewing gum, which tastes sweet but is very low in calories. Sweet fruits and vegetables like bananas and carrots may also help to satisfy you.

As with aversions, you will probably have cravings that are entirely personal to you. My main failing in this regard was an unquenchable hunger for cold rice pudding. For a period of some weeks when I was ill it became an important feature of my diet because I could not stand the thought of other foods. I was a little unsure as to whether this was a good thing at first, because of all the sugar and fat it contained. Then I reasoned that it had to be better than no food at all, and ate it to my heart's content. Just to satisfy my conscience about healthy eating, I made it with brown rice to keep up my fiber intake. As a general rule, satisfy your cravings where possible, but bear in mind your overall diet and do not allow excesses of sugar, fats or stimulants to continue for long.

Your Overall Diet

Your overall diet plan should provide enough of every type of food to fulfill your body's needs. Don't forget that even though you are doing very little, your body is working hard constantly to throw off your illness, so it is important that it gets enough food.

Many people find that a macrobiotic or whole food diet is helpful. These diets, high in natural nutrients, provide everything your body needs and eliminate most artificial additives. Also, the high fiber content in brown bread, brown rice, whole wheat pasta and so on, helps to maintain regularity in your digestive system and bowels, which can prevent constipation and other unwanted complications.

When to eat is another important question. Too many people eat little or nothing in the early part of the day, and make up for it later on with a big meal. This may suit you perfectly when you are healthy, but a fast-and-feast pattern is devastating when you are unwell. It places a strain on your entire system, one that you could well do without. Try to get into the habit of eating at least three small meals a day, at equally spaced intervals. By doing this you are regularly giving your body the fuel it needs to fight off the illness and function efficiently. You will soon notice the benefits of this regular eating routine. You will feel stronger, warmer and more alert and will be more resistant to a relapse.

EXERCISE

The simple answer to the question of exercise during illness is: don't. In the past doctors have often misguidedly ordered patients to exercise to relieve muscular pain and stiffness. It often makes the condition chronic. Even people who suffer little from the muscular problems associated with CFS will find that exercise is a sure and certain way to achieve a relapse.

When you are in a bout of illness, avoid exercise whenever possible. During convalescence, exercise becomes both necessary and beneficial.

As soon as you feel well enough to think about getting out and about, start to take a little exercise regularly. A daily stroll to the park or shops is great, but don't expect to be able to do this immediately. Start with trips into and around your own neighborhood. As your strength returns, gradually make more ambitious journeys. Always remain aware of your resources and never tire yourself to the point of inviting a relapse.

The benefits of exercise are many. Mentally, it gives you a lift, making you feel part of the world again. Fresh air and a change of scenery can do more to keep you alert and optimistic than any amount of therapy. Physically, the exercise helps to cleanse and tone your body, assisting it in getting rid of wastes effectively and maintaining a healthy balance. You will find that your sleep and appetite improve, and you will generally feel less feeble.

Avoid all violent or strenuous activities until you are sure, beyond a shadow of a doubt, that you can cope with them. Be prepared to stop whatever you're doing as soon as you feel that sinking, draining sensation that tells you your strength is ebbing. If in doubt, don't.

HEALING

The various names of spiritual healing, psychic healing and faith healing are all ultimately misleading. If healing needs any further description at all, place the word "natural" in front of it. Healing is the natural ability of one person to restore health in another.

Healing has existed for as long as mankind and is entirely independent of faith, psychic perceptions or spiritual beliefs. It is simply an exchange of energy from the healer to the patient that increases the patient's vitality. This leads to a quicker—sometimes instantaneous—recovery from illness or injury.

Most of us have experienced this type of energy exchange in everyday life. I am sure that you have come across people whose presence left you feeling uplifted, happy and full of energy. You have probably also met people who leave you feeling drained and dispirited. In each case, there has been an exchange of vital energy. The vital energy in each of us is not a static thing. It changes according to mood and environment, and it flows from person to person. Sadness, tiredness, depression and a host of other negative feelings allow our vital energy to drain away, and keep it from being replenished from the normal internal sources. When this happens, we unconsciously draw vitality from external sources in an attempt to regain our balance. These external sources are often other people.

Healers are people who either have a strong natural link with their own inner source of energy, or have worked and practiced to develop such a link. Once this link is functioning properly, the healer has an almost inexhaustible supply of vital energy that can be shared with anyone in need. This vitality can be directed to patients to help them overcome whatever internal or external factors have put them out of touch with their own source of strength. This then frees the natural healing powers of the patients' minds and bodies to correct any imbalances.

Healing is a very simple therapy. You only have to give the

briefest explanation of your problems to the healer, often none at all. Then he or she will start the treatment. Usually the healer will make contact with you by touching your shoulders, head or the problem area. Some healers prefer to hold their hands a few inches away from your body. As they start to send energy to you, you will probably feel a sensation of intense warmth spreading from their hands to your body. Occasionally, depending on the healer, the sensation might be one of coolness or tingling. The treatment usually lasts for a minimum of five minutes, and can go on for up to 15 minutes or longer if the practitioner feels you are badly in need of energy. During the treatment you will start to feel relaxed, happy and calm, and these feelings can stay with your for days after your session.

At various times I have been both healer and patient, though usually the former, and so I have a fairly comprehensive understanding of this therapy. I recommend it without hesitation to sufferers from any illness, regardless of its nature. I have never seen or heard of a case in which the patient did not benefit from the treatment in some way. The only limitation to the power of this vital energy is the skill, insight and experience of the healer. If you do not respond at first, find another practitioner.

Many times I have had people come to see me who looked awful—tense, drawn, tired and ill—but when they walked out after the treatment, their whole appearance had changed. In some cases, they actually seemed to be healthy again, and in every case their faces showed a glow of returning vitality. This outward change is only the echo of a more important inner healing. Within a period of hours, and sometimes minutes, even chronic conditions such as kidney failure, tumors and wasting diseases can be relieved by a proper application of the vital force of healing. Occasionally, they are cured outright. I know from experience that these "miracle" healings definitely do happen, but they are comparatively rare. Like most other therapies, healing has a cumulative effect over a period of time and a number of treatments. Expect to have to visit a healer a few times before big improvements become obvious. Little improvements may come about from the start, so the regular visit to your healer will probably become most enjoyable.

Healing is widely available, and very often healers will be willing to come to you if you are not able to travel to them. You may, however, have to pay their travelling expenses. Most faith and spiritual healers believe that their talent is a gift to be shared freely with the rest of mankind, and they do not charge for their services. Increasingly, though, people are coming to realize that the talent is purchased at the cost of long study and training, just the same as the skills of a therapist in any other field. And like other therapists, these practitioners have the right to charge patients for this skill and experience.

Charges vary widely. If you have the money to pay for healing, then it is probably wise to do so. This therapy is only as good as the individual practitioners, and a professional is more likely to be effective than a well-meaning amateur. It is not uncommon to find healers who give their services freely and are dedicated to high ideals, but who lack any real talent or training for healing. Persevere in your search for a reputable and able practitioner. When you find an effective healer the benefits to your health will be immediate and striking.

HERBALISM

Herbal medicine is best described as the art and science of restoring health by using remedies originating from plants. These remedies, referred to as herbs though they can come from any type of plant, are in many cases just as powerful as orthodox drugs but free from the toxic side effects of much drug therapy. Many qualified physicians are now studying herbalism to use alongside or instead of orthodox drugs.

There are records of this type of medicine being in use since at least 1500 B.C., so it is certainly one of the best established of alternative therapies. However, it is also the most complex, and treatment for serious complaints should be left exclusively to the professional practitioner.

When selecting an appropriate treatment for you, herbalists may look first at your symptoms, but they will also examine your temperament and mental state. The medicine they prescribe will take all of these factors into account. This means that treatment will vary widely from person to person, so it is of little use to suggest here which herbs might be beneficial to you.

Qualified herbalists can be difficult to find, and pursuing a course of treatment can be expensive. If you have had success with other plant-based therapies (aromatherapy, Bach flower remedies, etc.) it could be worth your while to try out this type of treatment. Ask in your local healthy food store whether they can refer you to a good local herbalist, or check the ads in health magazines. Herbalism should be quite safe to use in combination with the other therapies, but if you are also receiving homeopathic treatment or taking any other course of treatment, let all your therapists know exactly what you are doing.

HOMEOPATHY

Homeopathy is sometimes hard for people to accept as a valid system of medicine, for two reasons. The first is that its basic theory is completely opposed to medicine as we know and understand it. For example, a traditional (or allopathic) doctor will usually prescribe drugs that counteract the symptoms the patient is experiencing: If you have a fever, the doctor will give you something to cool you down. This seems perfectly logical and straightforward. A homeopathic doctor would approach the problem from the opposite direction. Instead of prescribing a cooling medicine, he would give you a tiny dose of a substance which in large quantities would cause the type of fever you are experiencing. This makes homeopathy difficult to understand for people brought up on allopathic principles of treatment.

The second reason for the lack of acceptance of homeopathy is the medicines themselves: The more they are diluted, the stronger they become. In many common preparations the original substance has been diluted to the point where the final tablet contains only one part per million of the substance. As we are all trained to think that power is measurable by its quantity or volume, this process of dilution seems to be counterproductive. However, before you dismiss this therapy out of hand, note these two facts: Homeopathy has been in existence since the 18th century and is one of the most widely available and consistently popular of all alternative therapies. We may not know how or why it works, but hundreds of thousands of people have found that it does.

Drawn from the animal, vegetable and mineral kingdoms, homeopathic remedies are thoroughly tested before they are approved for use. There are hundreds, or perhaps thousands, of these approved remedies and more are being discovered all the time. This means that homeopathic practitioners have a vast number of potential remedies at their fingertips. To make their choice they will require detailed descriptions of all your symptoms, and they will also take into account your temperament and, if applicable, your occupation, lifestyle and daily habits. This can make examinations hard work for the patient, but they are usually worthwhile. Most people who have persisted with homeopathic treatment report major or minor benefits, and they vary from person to person.

Although all homeopathic treatments are completely safe, it is such a complex system that selecting your own remedies is really out of the question. Most sizeable towns have at least one homeopathic doctor, so keep asking around until you find one in your area.

HYDROTHERAPY

The term "hydrotherapy" covers a vast range of techniques, all of which feature water as the main therapeutic agent. Many of these techniques are complicated and/or expensive, but two are appropriate for home use and can help all CFS patients. The first and most important is the hot bath.

The Hot Bath

Technically the temperature for a hot bath can be anywhere from 100°F upwards. In practice, you will want to have the water a lot warmer than that. The main benefit of a hot bath is the sweating it induces, and 100°F is too cool to do much good. However, having the water too hot is counter-productive. Remember that you are going to be in the bath for at least ten minutes and perhaps for as long as an hour, so select a temperature that will be comfortable over this period of time.

Having prepared your bath, the only other thing you have to do is get in and enjoy it. Wallow in the water, moving it around all parts of your body. Immerse yourself totally if possible—if not, then dip all parts regularly. Once you have started to sweat, relax until you feel you have had enough. When you get out, dry yourself well and wrap up to keep from getting chilled. Try to cool off gradually, always resting for at least an hour afterward. It is best to bathe in the evening so that you can fall into bed when you have cooled off a bit. A glass of water before bed is an excellent idea, to make sure you replace the fluid lost through sweating.

The first benefit of a hot bath is the obvious one. You get hot. This must not be underestimated. If you have been suffering from coldness, the relief of warmth is a blessing in itself. Apart from this, the bath will improve your circulation, bring you to a state of deep relaxation, and enable your body to sweat out many toxins and wastes produced by the disease. Sweating in a bath seems to help prevent the recurrence of night sweats and fevers. Generally, you will find that a hot bath reduces most of your symptoms to a noticeable degree and makes you feel better all over.

Combining the hot bath with other therapies is an excellent idea. Herbs and minerals added to the bath have an immediate effect as you can easily absorb them through the open pores of the skin. Personally, I find aromatherapy the best and simplest addition to hydrotherapy. The two combine luxuriously, enhancing each other enormously. It gives a whole new meaning to the idea of bathing.

Russian, Turkish, and sauna baths have exactly the same therapeutic effect as hot baths. If you have not tried these more exotic baths before, it is wise to stay in them for short periods only during your first few visits. You can gradually extend the length of your stay in subsequent visits, when you have adjusted to the intense heat.

The Neutral Bath

The second hydrotherapy technique of use to CFS sufferers is the neutral bath. As the name suggests, this is a bath of neutral, or blood, temperature. The main benefit of this type of bath is the deep relaxation it produces. It eliminates mental and physical tension and fatigue. Neutral baths can and should last longer than hot baths, so remember to keep adjusting the temperature so that you don't get too cold. Adding herbs, minerals or essential oils increases the therapeutic value.

The Alternating Bath

There is one other hydrotherapy technique that may be of use to some patients. If you have severe muscular pain and the swelling that sometimes accompanies it, then alternating baths will probably help you. The technique is perfectly safe and simple, but it can be quite a shock to the system as it relies on alternating hot and cold water in rapid sequence.

If it is your legs that require treatment, sit on the edge of the tub with your legs inside it. If any part of your upper body has to be treated, it will probably be simpler to undress completely and sit in the tub.

Once you are comfortable, start the treatment by running hot water over the affected muscles. Using a shower head for this is the best way, but quickly pouring bowls of water works almost as well. The water should be as hot as you can comfortably bear. After two, or at most three, minutes of hot water, switch immediately to very cold water and run this over the affected part for 30 seconds. Then switch back to hot again for another two to three minutes, followed by cold again, for 30 seconds. Repeat the hot/cold sequence once more to complete the process.

This treatment will reduce swelling and inflammation rapidly. Some patients report that it also reduces pain considerably for reasonable periods of time.

All of these hydrotherapy techniques are completely safe for regular home use. They will combine well with any other therapies.

HYPNOSIS AND AUTOHYPNOSIS

Many people still hold the outdated idea that hypnotists are Svengali-like characters whose only aim in life is to reduce the entire population to helpless zombies. Nothing could be further from the truth. The vast majority of hypnotists are responsible professionals who have mastered an excellent technique for helping people to help themselves.

Hypnosis can be defined as an altered state of consciousness in which the subject's logical, critical mind is bypassed. This state can be achieved only with the subject's consent. At all times you remain aware of and in control of your responses.

Being in a hypnotic trance is rather like being on the borderland between sleep and waking. You feel warm and comfortable and drowsy. While in this state your logical mind fades into the background, so you are very uncritical of anything you hear. If the hypnotist says, "You are feeling well. You are feeling strong. You feel no pain," then your mind accepts this as the truth. Because your critical faculty is "sleeping," you truly believe the ideas suggested to you by the hypnotist. Once your mind has fully accepted the suggestion that you are well and fit, you immediately start to feel better. This mind over matter effect is very real. Through the use of hypnosis your own unconscious becomes a strong ally in your struggle for health. By having the right suggestions accepted by the unconscious you can reduce or eliminate all of your symptoms.

Regular visits to a hypnotist can prove time-consuming and expensive, but if you already know from experience that hypnosis works for you, then it is a worthwhile investment. Alternatively, you can learn to hypnotize yourself quite quickly and cheaply, and produce excellent results in the privacy of your own home.

Autohypnosis, as self-hypnosis is called, is easy to learn from books and tapes. Once you master the basic techniques you can prepare hypnotic suggestions that will get your unconscious mind working to eliminate particular problems. It will probably take a little time and effort to get it right, but even when you are just starting to practice, you will benefit from the therapy. One of the by-products of the hypnotic state is mental and physical relaxation. This relaxation is extraordinarily helpful. You come away from it feeling as though you have just had a deep and refreshing sleep.

Unfortunately, hypnosis does not work for everyone, and as a therapy it is only as good as the practitioner who uses it. So, try autohypnosis first, preferably from a tape. If this is helpful, consider consulting a practitioner. They are widely available and advertise in most magazines and newspapers, but ask among your friends for a personal recommendation. Hypnosis or autohypnosis is safe in combination with any other therapy, and is enhanced by meditation and yoga exercises (see pages 88–89 and 102–105).

KINESIOLOGY

The techniques of this therapy are most widely known under the name "Touch for Health," which was devised by chiropractors for use by lay people. It is perhaps the simplest method of preventive health care available.

"Touch for Health" is not used for diagnosing or treating specific illnesses. It is used to discover and correct bodily imbalances of any kind. Correcting imbalances ensures that the body functions well and is able to heal itself. The simplest testing procedure indicates those parts of the body that are not working efficiently and suggests which thoughts, environmental influences or substances are responsible for the imbalance. It can show you which things will best return your body to a state of natural harmony.

Anyone can learn to administer the test procedure. The theory is that each of the 12 major body systems—stomach, lungs, pancreas, etc.—is closely related to certain muscles. Any system that is weakened or diseased will show as a weakness in the related muscles. Therefore, testing the muscles for simple physical strength gives a clear indication of internal functions.

What is really remarkable about this technique is the way in which you discover what has caused the imbalance and select a cure for it. A weak muscle will immediately grow weaker if you place a substance in your mouth that the body finds harmful. Conversely, the muscles will immediately strengthen if you place a beneficial substance in the mouth. This sounds quite straightforward, but you really have to experience the dramatic effect to comprehend fully how effective this technique can be. Within minutes you can test all the foods in your diet and find out which are harmful and which are helpful. You can also find out which vitamins, diet supplements, dietary changes or any other form of treatment will help you. You can use this technique to demonstrate clearly your internal reaction to absolutely anything. For CFS patients, knowing which things are acting against the body and weakening it can help to prevent or cure the relapses that occur from time to time, seemingly out of the blue.

Although it is possible to learn this technique from books, it is far better to attend one of the short instructional courses held regularly all over the country. Under the guidance of a trained instructor you will see the technique come to life in an amazing way. The basic course does not qualify you to practice as a therapist, but it does give you enough information to use the technique on friends and family. Unfortunately you cannot test yourself, so you will have to arrange for a friend to help you out with self-diagnosis. After you have shown your friends what can be done with this therapy, you will probably have people lining up to be tested; so arranging for one of them to test you in return should be no problem.

If you want to try this technique without going through the basic course, try to find a qualified practitioner near you. They may be difficult to find as they rarely advertise. Ask around, particularly in your local health food store. They may know of a practitioner in your area.

MASSAGE

A good massage stimulates the muscles just as effectively as a workout, so it's a good idea to treat massage with the same caution as exercise.

For people whose symptoms include muscular pain, massage is a definite "Don't." Although it may help to relieve pain at first (but certainly not always), it will cause the symptoms to become more intense in the following hours or days. It can even cause them to degenerate into a chronic condition.

If you suffer little from muscular pain and were receiving regular treatments from a masseur before your illness, it may be helpful to continue. During the massage you may find that particular areas or muscles feel tender. If so, ask your masseur to avoid these areas altogether.

If you have never had a massage before, then don't try this therapy during a bout of illness. In convalescence, if you are free of all muscular problems, it may be helpful.

The main benefits of massage are relaxation and stress relief, though it also helps with circulation and lymph drainage. It is widely available and can be combined with aromatherapy and hydrotherapy with excellent results.

MEDITATION

Strictly speaking, this is a discipline rather than a therapy, but because it has distinct therapeutic effects it deserves to be mentioned here.

Basically, meditation is the art of making the mind still. You let go of all the thoughts and feelings, hopes, fears and desires that occupy your mind so that it becomes peaceful and calm. This switching off of all day-to-day agitations of thought produces physical, mental and emotional relaxation. You emerge from the meditative state feeling renewed—calm, strong, refreshed and in control.

The only drawback with meditation is that it can be difficult to learn. Many people find that just as they achieve a degree of stillness, an idea appears from nowhere and their mind chases after it in fast and furious thought. Only patience and perseverance can cure this problem. There are no short-cuts to mastery of this technique. Every time your mind dashes off in a new direction, gently but firmly end the thought and return your mind to the stillness, which is empty of all thought, is very difficult to hold on to. If this is the case, select one thought or feeling to concentrate on and keep returning to it during practice periods. Concentrating on one thing only is a stepping-stone to concentrating on nothing. At this stage many people find that concentrating on their breathing is an excellent aid, while others prefer to focus their attention on an imaginary flower, a ball of light or any other comfortable image.

Trying to learn to meditate while in a bout of illness complicates the whole process. If you want to learn, wait until you are reasonably free of all mental symptoms. This will give you the best chance of succeeding quickly and well. However, recognize the fact that it is going to be weeks or months before you feel able to meditate easily, and be prepared to invest the necessary time and energy.

Once you have mastered the basics you will find that meditation is an ongoing process. The more you do it, the more you get from it. Mental and physical problems fade away as the meditation brings you into contact with deeper and deeper levels of your own mind. Eventually, you reach the point of feeling that while meditating you are in touch with the very center of your being. This releases a flow of strength and vitality that has to be felt to be believed.

Once you master meditation it will stand you in good stead for the rest of your life. In time it will balance and strengthen all the subtle energies of mind, body and spirit, paving the way for good health. "In time" is, unfortunately, the operative phrase. As a therapy, meditation is all about long-term goals and benefits, so it is best to consider this as a background therapy and seek other treatments for more immediate relief.

REFLEXOLOGY

Reflexology, which is simply massage of the hands and feet, has become one of the most popular alternative therapies now that different systems of medicine have caught the imagination of the public at large. Zone therapy, as this treatment is also called, is used as a means of bringing the patient back to a harmonious state of mind and body. Reflexologists believe that health is a direct result of this harmony, which cannot exist if any part of the intricate mechanism that is a human being is maladjusted.

No one can say for sure how or where the reflex method originated. One of the most popular theories is that it came to the West from China, where it existed alongside and was used with acupuncture. The fact that there are several important similarities between these two therapies tend to support the theory of an oriental origin, but reflexology is also known to have been used by the natives of Kenya and by some American Indian tribes. Whatever its origin, reflexology is simple and safe. It involves you in your own healing; it is an excellent diagnostic tool and equally effective as a preventive and a curative therapy.

The theory of reflexology is very straightforward. Every part of the body is linked, via the nervous system and the subtle energies, to a particular area of the hands and feet. When this area is stimulated by massage, the corresponding organ is affected. This is considered a natural reflex, hence the name. The fundamental therapeutic principle is one of releasing tension, thus bringing about a full blood flow to the dis-eased parts, but the massage also stimulates the subtle energies to revitalize and repair the affected area.

Because this reflex link works both ways, ill-health in any part of the body shows clearly in the corresponding reflex zone on the hand or foot. A skillful reflexologist can often diagnose problems before they are fully formed in the body, which is an invaluable aid in preventive health care. Whenever an organ is not functioning correctly, the associated reflex zone will become tender and sensitive to pressure. The discomfort varies according to the severity of the problem, so the practitioner often needs the patient's feedback about changes in the nature or strength of the discomfort. As soon as the pain in a particular area eases off, the corresponding organ is back in a state of good health.

Reflexology can aid CFS patients in a number of ways. It always produces relaxation, which amounts to a therapy in itself, and it helps most of the bodily systems to function efficiently. Digestion and the elimination of wastes are easily normalized by zone therapy, as are lymph drainage, breathing and circulation. Other benefits (there can be many) vary according to both patient and practitioner.

Finding a practitioner is simple as they are widely available, but finding a good one can be more problematic. Ask whether the practitioner has been trained in either the Ingham or the Bayly technique, as these are the most effective forms of the therapy. The only other guideline that is of any use is experience. If your session of reflexology is painful or leaves you feeling drained or ill, find another practitioner. A good practitioner is often sensitive enough to be able to establish a strong rapport with his or her patients, so feeling comfortable and at ease with the therapist is sometimes an indication that the therapy will eventually help you. Benefits should be noticeable from the first session onwards, and they will accumulate over a period of time with each subsequent session.

Reflexology is very simple, but the reflex zones themselves are quite complex. If you wish to invest some time and energy in learning the basics of the technique, you will be able to treat yourself on a daily basis or whenever you feel the need. Even if you would prefer to treat yourself, however, I recommend at least one session with a professional practitioner so that you can see and feel how it works in practice. This could make a vital difference to your newly acquired skills, as there is no way in which a book can explain the sensitivity that a good practitioner possesses.

This therapy is perfectly safe and compatible with all others. I have found that combining it with aromatherapy or healing produces particularly striking results.

RELAXATION

Since I have noted again and again the benefits of relaxation, it seems sensible to offer a relaxation technique so that you can try this simple therapy for yourself.

Lie on your back on the floor, and breathe in and out deeply a few times, just to prepare yourself. Then focus your attention on the toes of your right foot. Become aware of your toes as intensely as possible. Then breathe in deeply and clench your toes as tightly as you can, tensing up all the muscles. Hold this for a second; then breathe out slowly, relaxing your toes at the same time. Repeat this with the toes of the left foot. Return your attention to your right foot. Breathe in deeply and clench the muscles of the whole foot as tightly as possible. Hold this for a second, then breathe out and relax. Repeat this for the left foot. Now progress slowly up the body doing exactly the same thing to every muscle. Start with the calves, then progress to the thighs, the lower back, the stomach, the upper back, the chest, the arms, the forearms, the hands and fingers and finally the neck, scalp and face. Remember to breathe deeply as you tense and relax the muscles.

Doing this exercises properly will produce a sensation of warmth and heaviness in your muscles, and you will feel comfortably relaxed all over. You can combine this technique with any other therapy in perfect safety. Obviously, if you are suffering from severe muscular problems, don't try this method of relaxation. Instead, experiment with hydrotherapy, autohypnosis or yoga breathing as a basis for relaxation.

Many people do not fully realize the role that tension plays in illness. A tense body cannot heal itself effectively. Tension inhibits most of the body's systems, including circulation, lymph drainage, digestion, elimination of wastes, immune responses, recuperation and regeneration. The vicious circle of illness that produces tension that maintains illness that produces more tension has to be broken if the patient's natural healing mechanisms are to get the chance to overcome the disease. Therefore, regular relaxation is essential for health of both body and mind and should be included in any routine of therapy.

ROYAL JELLY

Thanks to the ever increasing popularity of this health and beauty treatment, many people now know that royal jelly is a thick off-white liquid produced by bees to feed their queen. What is less well-known is the phenomenally wide range of illnesses and complaints that can be alleviated with regular doses of this substance. Royal jelly is already known to be one of the most nutritious natural foods ever discovered, and reports of scientific investigations into its effects suggest that it is also one of the most potent natural medicines.

In the early days, research into this substance was painfully slow. Royal jelly is only produced in tiny amounts at certain times of year, so collecting enough for experimentation was an arduous task. Since the 1960s, scientific and medical interest, coupled with increased public demand, has encouraged bee-keepers to develop new techniques that trick the bees into producing much larger quantities of royal jelly (causing no harm to the bees). Now that royal jelly is freely available, there is a constant flow of new and exciting reports about its effects on the human system.

For many years we have been aware that royal jelly increases fertility and virility; improves the quality of hair, skin and nails; cleanses the blood; improves circulation and aids the efficient disposal of body wastes. The new reports being issued now show that it has an even more dramatic effect: It is an effective treatment for heart disease; it reduces cholesterol levels and prevents blocked arteries; it prevents and cures stomach ulcers and every other stress-related complaint; it is one of the most efficient natural disinfectants and has anti-fungal and anti-microbial properties; it can relieve even the most severe arthritic and rheumatic conditions; it is a potent diuretic; it improves the absorption of nutrients; it is an effective treatment for depression and neurotic states; it relieves eczema and most other skin complaints; and finally, to bring this list to a very premature end, it has been shown to be effective against cancer in mice, though no human trials have yet been reported.

With an immense weight of scientific evidence in support of royal jelly, it is surprising that it is still largely ignored by the medical profession. Part of the reason for this lack of acceptance is that we actually know very little about how royal jelly works. In fact, we do not even know entirely what it is made of. Analysis shows that 96 percent of the substance is composed of an effective combination of vitamins, minerals and amino acids, all of which are necessary for good health. The other four percent is a mystery that continues to defy analysis.

Another reason it is not used by the medical profession is that its effects are not consistent. Doctors are trained to expect that a drug will affect the great majority of individuals in the same way. Royal jelly does not do this. It affects each individual differently, according to their own needs, harmonizing and balancing their mental and physical systems. If it is given to a patient with high blood-pressure, it brings the blood-pressure down. If it is given to a patient with low blood-pressure, it pushes the blood-pressure up. In every case it normalizes the body, bringing natural functions to a peak of efficiency. Doctors seem reluctant to accept a treatment that acts differently according to the needs of the individual patient.

The doubts of the medical profession could be accepted as logical if royal jelly were a potentially dangerous treatment, but it is not. It is a safe, gentle, natural remedy that has never been known to cause any unpleasant side-effects. This being the case, you would imagine that doctors would be delighted to have found such an effective treatment for such a wide range of common ailments. I hope that as the evidence continues to mount, more doctors will put aside their preconceived ideas of what a drug is and how it should work, and accept royal jelly as a valid and valuable addition to their armory of treatments.

For CFS patients, royal jelly can help in a variety of ways. Among the most important are relief from muscular problems, increased energy and stamina and greater mental alertness. Many other symptoms respond equally well. In my own case I experienced a dramatic lessening of muscular pain, and over a period of weeks I regained a degree of mental clarity that I had not experienced since the illness started. I have seen people who were confined to bed or a wheelchair up and around again in a matter of weeks. One woman, who had been in constant pain for four years, was soon free of major difficulties and told me, "I keep thinking that I mustn't do things because of the pain, and then I remember that my legs don't hurt anymore. It's marvelous!" The vast majority of patients who have tried it report great physical and mental improvements.

If you decide to treat yourself with royal jelly, be prepared to give it an extended trial. For a normal healthy person using royal jelly as a preventive measure, it can take up to three months for this gentle natural substance to work its way into the system fully and start to produce results. For those of us who have been weakened by long-term or chronic sickness, it can take longer. Taking a higher dosage than normal can speed up the effects of the therapy, but otherwise persistence is the key word. Within the first two months you should begin to notice some improvements, no matter how small; these are a sign that eventually royal jelly will bring you greater benefits.

One other thing to note: During the first few days of your treatment you may actually feel worse. Royal jelly acts as a cleanser, helping the body to eliminate all wastes and toxins. As these toxins are cleared through the system and removed once and for all, your symptoms may get worse briefly. However, this takes only a few days, and then your body is free of all the poisonous by-products of the illness. This leaves you much more capable of being healed, so the brief period of worsening is not really a drawback.

Simple, safe and effective, royal jelly treatment is fully compatible with all other therapies. It is widely available through health food stores, but be careful which brand you buy; they are not all equally effective. When I am asked to recommend the best I suggest Regina Royal Jelly Ltd. The royal jelly in their products is pure, fresh and unprocessed. It comes only from beehives situated in remote regions of China where the air is pure and the crops are free of poisonous insecticides and fertilizers. If you have any difficulty buying Regina products in your area, you can write to the manufacturer for the address of your local supplier. Alternatively, you can order a supply of royal jelly directly from the company. The address of Regina is Elstree Way, Borehamwood, Hertfordshire WD6 1JD, U.K.

At the time of this writing Regina is carrying out medical tests of its royal jelly products against CFS. So far all of the trial participants have noted benefits of one sort or another and there is generally a feeling of great optimism. If you would like to try royal jelly, drop a line to the company to find out the results of the tests. They will be able to send you more information about royal jelly and to suggest which of their products would be most suitable for use in your particular case. When the tests have ended, they will also be able to tell you what is the most effective dosage, and so forth.

TISSUE SALTS

Tissue salts, or biochemical remedies, as they are more formally known, were developed by Dr. Wilhelm Schuessler in the last century. The remedies are each composed of a natural mineral that is necessary for the proper functioning of cells in the human body.

The theory that deficiencies of minerals in the cells could cause an overall disturbance of health became the life's work of Dr. Schuessler. His research led to the discovery of five principles:

1. Disease does not occur if cell activity is normal.
2. Cell activity is normal as long as all necessary nutrients are available.
3. The human body requires minerals as cell nutrients.
4. Mineral deficiencies will prevent the cell from functioning normally.
5. Individual cells, and therefore the whole metabolism, can be revitalized by correcting mineral deficiencies.

The doctor isolated 12 minerals that are necessary for

health, and used the homeopathic principle of trituration to form tablets that included a tiny dose of each mineral. All of the 12 tissue salts are completely safe and can be taken alone or in combination with other salts or therapies without any fear of side-effects.

In this therapy it is the predominant symptoms that point to the salt or salts necessary. For CFS patients, for example, tissue salt number 6 (Kali Phos) would be indicated in cases of nervous tension, depression and general debility; whereas muscular weakness would suggest the use of tissue salt number 1 (Calc Fluor). In addition to these two remedies, tissue salt number 4 (Ferr Phos) relieves muscular pain, and number 10 (Nat Sulph) can help in thrush and *Candida* infections. The other salts may also be suitable for individuals, but the four I mentioned are reliable aids for most CFS patients.

The benefit of this therapy is its simplicity and availability. You can buy the tablets in almost all health food stores and in some drugstores. The tablets are easy and pleasant to take, but follow the instructions carefully.

The drawback of this therapy is that lengthy treatment may be necessary before improvements are noticeable, especially if your condition is chronic or you have been ill for years. Of course, a speedy reaction to the treatment is possible, but it's best to consider this another background therapy.

VITAMINS AND DIET SUPPLEMENTS

VITAMINS

Several newspapers have reported stories of CFS patients recovering by taking large doses of one vitamin or another. Those who experience dramatic recoveries with this therapy seem to be a very small minority, but it does seem to have a helpful effect.

Unless we have a perfectly balanced diet every day, from time to time we all suffer from shortages of vitamins. There is no doubt that this is harmful if it continues over a long period of time. For CFS patients this is one more thing that can provoke the illness, even in the short term. Vitamins are essential for the proper functioning of all bodily systems. Without them—even for a short period—the body is weakened and can no longer defend itself properly against any illness. Making sure that your intake of food includes sufficient vitamins is a simple way to ensure that your body has everything it needs to function efficiently.

If your diet includes plenty of fresh foods (fruit, vegetables, meat, fish, etc.) which have not been processed or overcooked, then in all probability you are getting an adequate supply of vitamins. As insurance, however, it's a good idea to take daily multivitamin capsules. You can buy these from any health food store or drugstore.

Some people, myself included, have found it helpful to take a greater than normal amount of certain vitamins— particularly vitamin C and the B group, especially B_6. It is possible that CFS somehow increases your need of these vitamins, and it is quite safe to take them regularly. A good way to boost your vitamin B intake is to take a daily supplement of brewer's yeast, but take care. If you suffer from thrush or other *Candida* problems this may cause difficulties and you should try a yeast-free supplement instead.

Recent research in Canadian hospitals indicates that the vast majority of illnesses can be helped by increasing the patients' intake of vitamin C. The researchers gave every patient in a certain hospital high daily doses of this vitamin, and monitored their progress, comparing them with patients in another hospital who received no additional vitamins. The results were quite amazing. Relief from all sorts of problems was recorded, and recovery times were cut dramatically. In past experiments, even people suffering from incurable diseases have responded incredibly well to this therapy. This suggests that anyone who is ill would do well to keep a close eye on vitamin intake. However, if you are thinking about experimenting with extremely high doses of vitamins be sure to work under the supervision of a qualified physician.

Minerals

Minerals, too, are necessary for a healthy body, but in much smaller amounts than vitamins. Certain minerals can be lacking from your diet for any number of reasons, including your geographical location. Making sure that your diet is supplemented with minerals, or trace elements as they are called, is a sensible preventive measure. Multi-mineral tablets are readily available, and they can often be bought combined with multivitamins. This simplifies the whole therapy into a one-tablet-a-day regimen.

There is a growing awareness that a few specific minerals can have a dramatic effect on health. Two minerals in particular have been mentioned in connection with CFS. Germanium and selenium are currently being researched quite extensively because there is reason to believe that they strengthen the body's immune system, helping it to heal itself of disease. Tests have been carried out using these substances, and although the results are not always conclusive, they do suggest that in some cases a daily dose of one of these minerals can promote a speedy recovery. As long as you follow the dosage instructions carefully, these diet supplements should be perfectly safe, so it may be worthwhile for you to try them. However, these immune-supportive substances are a relatively new approach to treatment and as yet we do not know exactly how or why they work. If you think that an immune-supportive supplement is a good idea, try royal jelly first (page 93). It supports the immune system in many ways, is perfectly safe, and provides essential vitamins and minerals in an easily absorbed form.

A number of other diet supplements have been tried by CFS patients. In some cases they report substantial improvements; in others, no improvement at all. As the response to these supplements is so varied, I cannot really recommend them fully. However, they seem to work for some people so you may want to give them a short trial. If you have tried any of these supplements before for other ailments and found them successful, that is a good indication that they will probably help you to some extent in combating CFS.

Other Supplements

The first of these possible supplements is Evening Primrose Oil. It is sometimes sold as a remedy for pre-menstrual tension, but don't let that put you off. It seems to be beneficial in a number of ways—including having a strengthening and balancing effect on the nervous system—so this remedy may be helpful against the nervous disorders associated with CFS. Most people who have tried it continue to take it regularly, which is some indication that it is doing them good, but often they cannot put their finger on any specific improvement.

Ginseng is one of the more popular diet supplements. I have heard it praised quite highly, but again the people who like it find it difficult to express exactly what it does for them. As it is generally known for its tonic properties, it is reasonable to assume that it will harmonize the body, allowing it to heal itself more effectively. I would imagine that it also boosts your energy reserves, and so may be an antidote to the weakness and tiredness that affects so many patients.

Garlic, both fresh and in capsules, is another remedy that

has achieved a degree of popularity. It is usually prescribed for problems of the heart, lungs or digestive system, so quite how it affects CFS is a mystery. Again, the improvements it brings tend to be minor, but some patients, particularly those with predominantly muscular symptoms, find it beneficial as a regular supplement. They recommend taking it in high doses, so it might be just as well to protect your social life by taking the deodorized capsules rather than the fresh plant.

Shark Liver Oil is a relatively new product on the market. As yet its properties are not fully understood, but there are claims that it is a powerful immune-supportive agent. It has been used in tests against certain types of cancer with some impressive results, but this research is definitely in its infancy. It will be many years before it is fully documented. CFS patients who have tried this supplement are quite complimentary about it, reporting a general overall lightening of symptoms. The degree of relief varies significantly from person to person.

All of the diet supplements mentioned here are safe to use as a regular daily therapy, but be sure to discuss any supplements you wish to take with your doctor. It is worth experimenting further in this field, to try to discover a supplement that really helps, but don't be disappointed if you have only minor successes. In most cases, diet supplements should be thought of as a background therapy.

YOGA

Yoga can be defined as the science of maintaining a healthy mind in a healthy body, and for centuries it has been known as a preventive therapy. It is also used increasingly in a remedial way to produce cures or alleviation of disease. Research in India and elsewhere has identified specific areas in which yoga practice, particularly hatha yoga, has alleviated illnesses. In many cases it leads to permanent cures. Some of these areas are very relevant to CFS patients—constipation, migraine, neck and back pain, nervous debilitation and depression.

Yoga is basically a philosophy, a way of thinking and a way of life. It embraces every aspect of existence—spiritual, emotional, mental and physical. It is a system of conscious evolution or self-improvement that has been cherished and embellished over the 6,000 years of its documented existence. The main reasons why people take up yoga are to reduce nervous tension, to slim down, or to become more agile physically and mentally. However, a study of yoga leads naturally to meditation, modifications of thought and behavior and a new realization of the purposes and processes of life. This holistic approach leads to better health and the eradication of physical and mental dis-ease.

The belief underlying yoga is that most ailments are caused by wrong posture, wrong diet and wrong mental attitudes. These imbalances are under the control of the student, or patient, exclusively and can only be corrected by the individual. Therefore it is up to the student to improve through the regular and proper practice of yoga techniques. The therapist, or teacher, is not in any way responsible for the student's success or failure. They are only there to help the student learn the techniques correctly, and to suggest which techniques might be best in any situation. Responsibility for the success of the therapy lies entirely with the student.

A typical hatha yoga class consists of exercises performed standing, kneeling, sitting, lying on the back, lying on the front and inverted. The exercises are performed slowly and gently, and should never cause any undue effort or strain. The aim of the exercises is to strengthen and improve the flow of subtle energies by flexing the whole body and by holding certain postures. Any strain or effort is counterproductive as it weakens or blocks energy flows rather than strengthen them. Along with the exercises the class will probably include a number of relaxation periods during which students are taught to relax completely, or perhaps an introduction to meditation.

After a properly conducted yoga session you should feel relaxed and at peace, both mentally and physically, with no pains from over-exertion, nor should you have any feeling of having performed well or badly compared with the other students. Yoga is totally noncompetitive. You go as far with each exercise as you comfortably can, and no further. As you master each posture and become able to perform it easily, the teacher introduces you to a new exercise or a new variation on the one you are doing, so that you are constantly putting the best effort you can muster into a series of increasingly taxing postures.

For CFS patients, yoga is partially exempt from the general rule about avoiding physical exercise. Under the guidance of an experienced teacher, yoga is probably safe for even a complete beginner with this disease. Experienced students with CFS can continue their practices, but should be prepared to drop back to simple exercises or to give up altogether during bouts of illness. As always, remain highly aware of your own state of health, and discontinue any exercises that affect you adversely.

One of the breath control, or *pranayama*, exercises of yoga is excellent for all ill people, regardless of the nature of their ailment. It aids breathing, circulation and digestion, and prevents constipation. It produces deep relaxation and mental clarity, removing all fatigue and tension. It is also perfectly safe for daily, or more frequent use.

Sit or lie in a comfortable position, making sure that your chest and stomach can move freely. Keeping your mouth closed, breathe in through your nostrils. Breathe in until your lungs are comfortably full of air and your stomach is pushed out. Then breathe out, pulling your stomach in until your chest deflates. Repeat this a few times to get the feel of it. Remember to breathe slowly and evenly, keeping your mouth closed.

Once you have got the feel of this deep breathing, start to count mentally while you breathe. Count slowly to four while you breathe in. Then hold your breath for the same count, by holding the muscles of your chest and stomach quite still. Then breathe out to a count of six, and again hold the muscles of your chest and stomach still for a count of four. Then repeat the whole exercise again, starting with the "in" breath. Continue for as long as you like, but do keep it going for at least several minutes. Remember to breathe evenly and slowly, and never hold your breath by closing your throat. Keeping the muscles of the chest and stomach still will prevent air from entering or leaving your lungs in a much more harmonious fashion.

This regular, rhythmic breathing is an excellent therapy. As you become more experienced with it and do not have to concentrate so hard on the counting, you will be able to feel the relaxation it produces. Five minutes of controlled breathing leaves you refreshed and invigorated. When the rhythm becomes easy to follow, you'll be able to do it at any time and in any situation, and it will always release a new flow of energy into your mind and body.

5

THE IMPORTANCE OF MENTAL ATTITUDE

The workings of the human mind are subtle and little known. We can only guess at the connections between mind and body, and at how these two aspects of self influence each other. The more we learn, the more it seems that mind and body form an indivisible whole, like two sides of a coin. For as long as life lasts mind and body are part of each other, acting and reacting as a single unit.

Accepting this truth about our basic nature means that we have to examine our attitudes towards health and illness. We can't consider either state as purely physical any longer. We have to realize that physical disease is always accompanied by, and is sometimes caused by, mental dis-ease. Therefore any attempt to cure a disease of the body must include curing the dis-ease of the mind as well.

Your own mind can be your strongest ally or your greatest enemy in the quest for well-being. If your thought patterns are of health, strength and optimism, your body will be influenced to respond with increased vitality, healing itself rapidly and well. If your thought patterns are despairing, fearful and pessimistic, every healing mechanism in your body will be sabotaged and true health may never be achieved. Learning to harness the power of your mind and to direct it into positive channels of health and growth is the quickest, safest method of preventing or curing any ailment.

The importance of mental attitude cannot be over-emphasized. Thinking the right things in the right way is the key to success in any situation. When the situation is illness and your own body is the monitor showing your success or lack of it in no uncertain terms, thinking correctly becomes a necessity. Too many people choose to remain unaware of their potential, accepting their mental habits and processes as an unchangeable facet of their being, completely beyond their control. But in just the same way that your body is always changing, functioning well or badly according to what you put into it, your mind is constantly changing too, adjusting its functions according to the diet of thoughts, ideas and expectations you feed it. Just as an adequate supply of good food will build an efficient and healthy body, an adequate supply of good thoughts will build an efficient and healthy mind. The healthy mind, one free of dis-ease, is a powerful influence in helping you overcome bodily disease. The diet of thoughts your mind needs to perform this healing is generally known as positive thinking.

Positive thinking releases a flow of energy into your mind and body. You feel stronger, healthier, more relaxed and more optimistic. If you persist in training your mind to follow positive thought patterns, the cumulative effect is enormous. You can literally feel yourself rising above the pain and weakness of disease. It is like rising up through the rain and clouds into a realm of pure air and sunshine.

Training yourself to think positively is fairly simple but it does require perseverance. Every time you feel yourself slipping into a negative attitude you have to make the effort to correct your thoughts, always concentrating on the positive, pleasant alternative. Instead of giving in to fears about your illness, you continually consciously reinforce your knowledge that you are getting better. Instead of feeling miserable because you cannot do the things you want, you concentrate on all the things you can do and allow yourself to feel pleasure at each small achievement. If you always make yourself look for the bright side of things you will soon find that no matter how depressing the situation, you can get something positive from it.

Rules of Positive Thinking

There are a few basic rules of positive thinking that you have to abide by if you want your mind to help you. The first is that it is useless to phrase a positive thought in a negative way. For instance, thinking, "I am not ill" will have very little effect at all because it stresses a negative: "I am *not* ill." The same idea expressed positively would probably come out as, "I am well" or "I am getting better." Both of these will be effective, because they are simple, direct, positive suggestions that your mind can take up and work on.

Another rule, and a very important one, is to let your imagination in on the act. When you tell yourself, "I am getting better," reinforce this by imagining how great life will be when you are healthy. Imagine yourself strong and alert, free of all symptoms, able to live a happy, healthy, normal life. It doesn't matter whether you imagine this in pictures or words or feelings or a combination of all of them, as long as you add all the details that are particularly relevant to you. If the thing you miss most is playing tennis or golf, imagine yourself on the court or fairway having a wonderful time. Whatever you most want to be able to do again should be the central focus of your imaginings, but don't forget the important little things as well—taking a stroll with someone special, visiting friends in the evening or having your family over to dinner. All of these things can be strong sources of positive thought.

The third and final basic rule is to get your emotions into the act. When you imagine yourself healthy and able, think about how that's going to make you feel. Will you be happy, triumphant, ecstatic, fulfilled? Let your emotions color in the picture you have imagined; then watch it come to life. Your emotions are the powerhouse of your mind. Positive thinking provides images of the reality that you are bringing into being, and it is positive feeling that fuels the process of change, moving you towards whatever you have imagined.

Daily Practice

On a daily basis it's a good idea to practice two types of positive thinking. The first, which I have described above, is very quick and pleasurable to do. Take a few minutes in the morning and a few at night to imagine and feel yourself healthy. After the first few days, when you are used to the technique and really have the "feel" of what you're doing, you will probably find that just the act of imagining health makes you feel better. The effects will build up day by day, becoming stronger and more tangible for as long as you keep thinking positively.

The second type requires more effort and does not produce such noticeable results, but it is effective in the long run and is a necessary support for the first type. It simply consists of being aware of your own thoughts. During bouts of illness it is very easy to slip into negative thought patterns. Simple things like washing up, making the beds or going shopping can become impossible, and it is natural to regret the fact that you cannot do any of these things.

If you listen carefully to your thoughts at this point, you will probably hear yourself saying something like, "Oh, I wish I could do that," or "I just can't do it. I feel too sick." These thoughts are natural, but they are also harmful. By repeating them you are reinforcing the ideas of "I can't" and "I am sick." When you find yourself in the midst of thoughts like these, stop immediately and replace them firmly with a more positive command, such as, "I will be able to do that soon," or "I am stronger every day." After a while, your unconscious mind will get the message that negative thoughts and negative phrases are unwelcome, and it will start to present ideas in more positive forms.

When this happens you'll know that your new, more positive phrasing of ideas has sunk down into the lowest levels of your mind. It is when your unconscious starts thinking habitually in positive ways that you get the most striking results. The two types of positive thinking I've described work together to make sure that your unconscious rapidly adopts new thought patterns that will work to your benefit.

There is one other technique of positive thinking that is very simple and effective: The affirmation. Detailed books have been written about this single technique, but in essence it boils down to this: Pick a positive, simple slogan for yourself and repeat it as often as possible. I am sure that everyone must have heard of the famous statement. "Every day in every way I am getting better and better." This is a brilliant example of the affirmation. It is a short, uncompli-cated positive thought expressed in simple terms. Inciden-tally, it makes a fine affirmation for CFS patients, but you may prefer to create one tailored to your own specific needs. Ideally, an affirmation should express the essence of every-thing you want your mind to help you achieve. Then regular repetition pushes the idea firmly into your mind at a level where it will influence you deeply. It is usually best to let your emotions help the affirmation by "feeling" its meaning once a day. Then repeat it to yourself, physically or mentally, every time you find yourself sliding backwards into doubt or negativity.

The Affirmation Spot

Some people believe that there is a simple addition you can make to your affirmation routine that will vastly improve results. I have known this technique as the affirmation spot.

The affirmation spot is easy to make and use. Get yourself a small piece of paper or cardboard, and on one side color in a circle about ¼-inch diameter. Use a nice bright color for the spot—red is ideal. When you finish, select a time and place that you know will be peaceful, so that you will have an uninterrupted five minutes to "charge" the spot.

Charging the spot is simplicity itself. Just look at it while you think of your affirmation. Say it to yourself mentally and physically, repeating it over and over again. Let your emotions feel the meaning of your slogan. Imagine how life will be when your affirmation has become reality. Try to make it an intensely positive experience. When you have finished, all that remains is to put your affirmation spot in a place where you will see it fairly often. By the stove or sink would perhaps be a good place for you, or over a mirror or on a coffee table. If you are at work, place the spot on a door or inside a drawer—anyplace in which you will see it at least three or four times a day.

The principle of this technique is that when you charge the spot, you concentrate on the simple image of the color circle, driving this image deep into your mind. Along with the image go all the thoughts and feelings conjured up by the affirmation. Afterwards, every time you see the spot you are reminded of the intense positive thought you used to charge the spot. This keeps your conscious mind working along the positive track expressed in the affirmation. More importantly, it continually prompts your unconscious, acting as a command to speed and strengthen the healing process. Recharging your spot once a week or so will maintain a high level of effectiveness.

Dealing with the Caregivers

Apart from the direct benefits to health of positive thinking, there are other desirable side effects. Most important of all is a renewal of your self-respect. Long-term illness can make you feel like a waste of space, a millstone around the neck of your family. Thinking positively helps you adjust to the fact that you must to some extent rely on others. Adjusting well to this fact takes a lot of pressure off you and the people who care for you, and allows everyone to be more optimistic.

Having the support of your family and friends is important. When you are in a bout of illness, they may be your only link with the world outside. Even when you are convalescent and able to get out and about on your own, the people around you are a valuable source of news, gossip and entertainment that keeps you in touch with normalcy. They are a breath of fresh air in a world that may have shrunk to the size of your own house or room.

Spare a thought occasionally for your caregivers because they are doing an extremely difficult job. They have watched you change from a normal human being to a withdrawn, unresponsive, dependent patient. Watching someone you care for go through a disease like CFS is a frightening experience. You instinctively want to protect your loved one, but there is absolutely nothing you can do to ease that pain. Very often the caregivers are as frustrated by the illness as the patient is.

Over a period of time this frustration can wear down the caregivers' understanding to the point where they seem to become unsympathetic. The constant pressure of not knowing what to do or how to help becomes unbearable. They would rather not be around the illness—and therefore the patient—any more. Not looking at the reality of a situation like this may relieve the feeling of helplessness, but it puts even greater pressure on the relationship between you if the caregivers have retreated emotionally.

It is your job as the patient to help your caregivers whenever and however possible. Obviously, when you are very ill there is little you can do to make their job easier. In convalescence, however, you have the opportunity to support the people who are supporting you. The most vital thing is to communicate with them. You may feel that you have little or nothing of interest to say, but say it anyway. Talking, even if it is only about the weather, reassures your caregivers that you are back in the land of the living. Tell them how your day has been, concentrating on all the little achievements. Talk with them about the news, or a book you are reading or their interests or hobbies. Make the effort to chat. It is the most basic form of human communication and it is immensely comforting.

Another way in which you can help your caregivers is to accept their support gracefully. It is very easy to get into the habit of feeling guilty about the demands and pressures you are putting on the people around you. This guilt stems from a feeling of inadequacy—you cannot do for yourself the things that you think you should be doing. Feeling this way can lead you to reject the help that people offer, or even to reject the people themselves. This creates a very unhappy atmosphere. For everyone's sake you need to overcome this guilt and treat your caregivers with the respect and courtesy that they deserve.

If people offer to help you with things that you cannot do for yourself, accept the help gracefully and express your thanks. If you find yourself getting caught up in feelings of guilt about accepting aid, tell yourself firmly that you need help at the moment, but you will soon be well enough to take care of yourself. This is not only good positive thinking, it is good practical thinking, too. You get the help you need, which makes you feel better; and your caregivers are able to express their concern by helping you, which makes them feel better. Remember that they are as frustrated by your illness as you are, and helping you is the only way in which they can feel as if they are doing something constructive.

Support Groups

Apart from friends and relatives, some people find that support groups can be helpful. As the name implies, these are local groups of patients who get together once in a while to compare notes and talk about anything relevant to CFS. Meeting other patients is often a good thing. You no longer feel so dreadfully alone in your fight against the illness, and there is a sense of camaraderie that can become the basis of some good friendships.

Unfortunately, there can also be a negative element about these groups. Some of them seem to focus exclusively on the pains and problems of the illness, which can be depressing. Most groups, however, approach the subject with a sense of humor, helping patients to laugh at themselves and find the bright side of difficult situations. These groups are also an excellent way of keeping in touch with new developments in research or treatment, as well as providing a good source of tips on how to cope with various aspects of the illness.

This exchange of information is the most important thing that goes on in support groups. Other patients can suggest therapies and techniques that you may find helpful, or tell you of energy-saving ways to go about necessary tasks. This makes you feel as though you have some ammunition with which to fight the disease, and that helps to keep you optimistic. Another benefit is that you always find people who have specific symptoms much more severely than you do, and this helps you to keep things in perspective and on a positive track.

Often the most valuable advice a newcomer receives from longer-term patients is this: Learn your own limitations. This is the most basic rule of living with CFS, and you ignore it at your peril. You need to develop an attitude of constant awareness of your energy levels. As soon as they start to drop to a degree where your symptoms could get worse, you must rest immediately. This regime of limitation can get incredibly frustrating, but if you do not enforce it, then the virus will, by making you ill every time you deplete your energy reserves.

Centered-With-Self

Living within the limits of your resources demands that you adopt an attitude that borders on selfishness. If you are out shopping, or in the middle of cooking dinner or entertaining friends when you feel your energy drop, you have to stop immediately and rest. Many patients intensely dislike being self-centered in this way. They feel that they are already causing enough problems for their friends and families without stopping dead in the middle of an outing or chore. However, it is essential that you do this when the need arises, so you might as well make up your mind to accept it as a temporary fact of life.

It helps if you stop thinking of this behavior as self-centered, and start thinking of it as "centered-with-self." This might seem like word play and of little practical value, but in fact it does help. By using the term "centered-with-self," you are removing all of the selfish, "me first" connotations that we associate with the term "self-centered." "Centered-with-self" is simply an acknowledgment that you must put your own needs first. That will, of course, work to everyone's benefit in the long run. By protecting yourself in the present you are preventing relapses and future complications that could keep you ill and disabled for months.

While it is very important to live sensibly and stay well within the bounds of your strength, it is also necessary that you do whatever you can. You may often find yourself in a situation where you are feeling up to doing something, but know that you will not have the stamina to finish the job. You might find yourself thinking, "If I can't finish it, then it's not worth starting." This is an understandable attitude, but a negative one. Always do the maximum that you safely can. If that means starting a job one day and finishing it the next, or the day after—that is fine. Making yourself do little bits and pieces has several good effects. The first is that the physical exercise, as long as it is not too strenuous, will act as a tonic, helping your body function efficiently. The second and most important effect is that the exercise will tone up your mind and give you a little glow of satisfaction at having achieved something. This helps you to stay positive and to maintain your self-respect.

Every little thing that you can do should act as a trigger for some self-satisfaction. Think of all these little things as stepping-stones back to health, each one bringing you a little closer to the day when you will be fully active. Use these little achievements to reinforce your positive thinking, keeping your thoughts firmly centered on health rather than illness.

Remember also to keep things in perspective. If you have been so ill that making a cup of tea seemed like a lifetime's work, then this has ceased to be a trivial thing. The first time you make a cup of tea without really thinking about it is a massive achievement, comparable to running a marathon or passing your driving test. Congratulate yourself on this big step forward; allow yourself to feel pleased and satisfied, and celebrate by getting out the danish or doughnuts to go with this momentous cuppa.

When you have only enough energy to do one thing per day, what should it be? Cleaning up? Spending time with your family? Taking a walk? If you can decide what to do, you have determined what your priority is and you should stick to it. Many of the things that we wish we could do in the course of a day are really very unimportant, so it is wise to decide what deserves your best efforts. Getting your priorities in order is a good way to make sure that you don't waste the little energy you have on meaningless pursuits. Look ahead to identify each day's major items, and plan your activities so that you are rested and refreshed when something important comes up. This will make you feel that you are coping with life more successfully and responding to those things that require your time and energy.

All of the things I have talked about in this chapter have to do with attitude. Developing the right attitude to your illness will reduce your suffering, make life easier for you and your caregivers and result in a quicker recovery. The wrong attitude can undo much of the good done by the therapies you undertake. Your thoughts are very powerful. Make sure that this power is working with you, not against you.

6

FOR THE CAREGIVERS

As I have pointed out, watching a close friend or loved one going through a disease like CFS is a trying experience. In the early stages, both patient and caregiver are frightened and worried about the cause of this ailment. Just as the patient unconsciously fears a fatal or degenerative disease, so do you, the caregiver. In this sense an accurate and speedy diagnosis is just as important for you as it is for the patient. During the later stages of the illness, the pressures on the patient tend to remain fairly constant, while the caregiver's pressures change and grow.

If you live with someone who has CFS, during the first few weeks and months of the illness the greatest pressures on you are going to be the practical ones—shouldering the burden of shopping, housework, cleaning, cooking and all the other activities that used to be performed jointly or by the patient alone. At first this extra workload is not too much of a problem. In a way, doing these extra tasks expresses your desire to help your disabled friend, mate, spouse, parent or offspring. In time, however, the burden can become very heavy indeed. You may be working to support the family, taking care of the children and maintaining a home; and far from offering any support or assistance, the patient is just another responsibility—another demand on your resources. Over a period of months, or even years if the illness is severe, you can find your sympathy and supportiveness ebbing away completely.

This practical burden is complicated by the emotional burden of the illness. When the patient is too ill to understand you or respond to you in any way, you feel totally cut off and unappreciated. When the patient is experiencing mood swings or depressions, you are unsure how to handle this new and strange personality. When the patient is in pain, confused and frustrated, you will bear the brunt of that anger, guilt, and sense of inadequacy. And overriding all this is your constant feeling of helplessness. In this situation it would not be at all surprising if you started to feel that you needed to get away not only from the illness, but also away from the person who is putting such demands upon you. The very thought of getting away can make you feel guilty of desertion.

Many marriages in which one partner is a patient have almost come to grief over this thorny problem. Maintaining high levels of care and sympathy for the helpless person who was once your spouse is nearly impossible, without certain adjustments. The major adjustment the caregiver must make is exactly the same as the one that must be made by the patient—learning to live with CFS.

Just as the patient must adjust to a new physical lifestyle, so must the caregiver: You need to allow more time for those extra chores, plan your time and energy wisely and decide what your priorities are and what can wait. Just as the patient must develop new positive mental attitudes and processes, so must the caregiver: You need to learn to think positively, maintain a degree of optimism and keep things in perspective. Just as the patient must rework his or her emotional responses, so must the caregiver: You need to learn to release negative feelings, focus on the good feelings that accompany every small achievement and consciously reinforce the image of a normal, happy, healthy lifestyle.

This book is about helping patients find the breathing spaces that help them to get away from the illness in order to refresh their minds and bodies. You, as the caregiver, must also allow yourself time to get away from the illness. Regularly pursuing your favorite sport or hobby is an excellent way to forget the illness for a while. Never feel guilty about going out and having fun while the patient is ill at home. Making sure that you forget all about the illness whenever you need to is good for everyone concerned. You will return refreshed in mind and body, more willing and able to care for the patient in a spirit of sympathy. Equally, the patient will fell less guilty about being a burden on you. Tying yourself down completely to the patient 24 hours a day is the fastest way to wear yourself out, destroying the strength and resilience that both of you need so badly. Consciously plan ahead to set aside fun times for yourself, to get away from all the limitations of CFS.

Any of the therapies mentioned in this book will be excellent for you to use as a preventive measure, safeguarding your own well-being. Some of the therapies can become a fun time you can participate in together. This shared activity will be beneficial to the health of both of you, and will also help to maintain the shared experience that helps keep a relationship growing. Going to see a healer together, or taking your royal jelly capsules every morning, or learning to meditate or experimenting with aromatherapy—all these can be used to enhance the bond between you and help to keep your relationship stable in spite of the illness.

These shared activities can be a lifeline for the patient. After being isolated for weeks by a thick fog of pain and confusion, hating yourself for being so feeble, having someone there who understands the limitations and can take you out of yourself for a while is wonderful. Once, when I was just coming out of a particularly bad bout of illness, a friend arrived one morning to take me on a so-called "mystery tour." In fact, there was not much mystery about it because she took me to a local woodland that I had known for years. She knew, though, that I had also loved it for years and that being there in the fresh air had always been wonderful therapy for me. We sat and talked in the sunshine for a while, and then she dropped me off at home. I was absolutely exhausted, but it was a good healthy tiredness. I slept well and awoke refreshed. The fact that my friend had involved herself in my therapy, and helped me in a very practical way, was a real tonic. It made me feel as though I had re-established contact with the human race.

Caring for anyone with a long-term or chronic illness is all about keeping up a degree of normalcy, sharing things in the way you used to. Of course, the things you share have to change because of the limitations of the illness, but the act of sharing can and should be maintained. This applies to friends of CFS patients as well as to live-in caregivers.

If you have a friend who is suffering from this debilitating disease, then you will find your friendship going through a very tough time. Most friendships are based on the things that people do together, and there is very little a CFS patient can do when ill or convalescing. Many patients, particularly those in the younger age groups, have found that their friends start to disappear from sight after the first few weeks of illness. This is unfortunate but understandable. It is during periods of convalescence and remission when the patient is alert enough to want and need human contact that the lack of friendly visits and phone calls becomes most noticeable. At this stage it can be very depressing to feel isolated and out of touch.

If you are a friend of a CFS patient, make the effort to stay in touch. A five-minute phone call can make an extraordinary difference. On many occasions during the course of my illness, I was too well to stay in bed sleeping, but too ill to do anything interesting or go out. At these times I would feel bored and listless, trapped inside the walls of my house. A phone call was an absolute godsend. The fact that someone had bothered to pick up the phone to find out how I was doing and to chat for a few minutes seemed like a real lifesaver—or a sanity-saver, at least.

Strangely enough, very often patients do not feel able to call their friends, no matter how bored or restless they feel. I can relate to that. After all, when you call someone what do you have to say—that you are still feeling awful and have not been anywhere or seen anyone? It doesn't feel right to inflict this bad news on a friend. You feel as though you're infecting others with your boredom and misery. If, on the other hand, others call you, it's much easier to gloss over your own situation and concentrate on talking about the callers. Chatting with healthy friends about their activities and thoughts can be a real high point in your day. It helps to establish that feeling of normalcy and contact with the real world.

Occasional visits are good for patients too, though they may not be terrifically entertaining for the visiting friend. If you want to see a CFS patient, your visit will be much appreciated—as long as you don't just turn up out of the blue. Unless you know very well how the patient is feeling, a surprise visit is not a good idea. When patients are in a period of illness, they often need to be left alone. If they are in convalescence, you might turn up when they need to be sleeping or resting. A phone call before you arrive is always a good idea. If you arrive at a bad time it can be awkward for all concerned. If patients are too embarrassed to explain the situation to you and to ask you to leave, it can lead to them over-exerting themselves because of your visit. Keeping in touch with patients fairly regularly is the best way to get an idea of the state of their health. You will soon be knowledgeable enough about their pattern of good and bad times to know when a visit would be most welcome.

Finally, the one thing a patient needs from friends and caregivers more than anything else is their optimism, their belief that in the not-too-distant future the patient will be back to radiant health. Because CFS is a long and severe illness, it is all too easy for patients to lose their sense of direction, their aims and their goals. In effect, they get lost in the illness and can no longer see any possibility of health. Having people around who believe in their ability to beat the disease is a constant help. It is like a signpost that always points in the right direction, encouraging the patient to take the next step, and the next—back to health.

CFS ORGANIZATIONS

The following is a partial list of CFS organizations. You may obtain information from them by sending a self-addressed stamped envelope with $.45 postage on it. The organizations will provide names of local support people and physicians, as well as general information.

In the United States

Chronic Fatigue Immune
Dysfunction Society
Community Health
Services
1401 East Seventh Street
Charlotte, North Carolina
28204

Chronic Fatigue Immune
Dysfunction Syndrome
Society International
Post Office Box 230108
Portland, Oregon 97223

Chronic Fatigue Syndrome
Association
919 Scott Avenue
Kansas City, Kansas 66105

Southern California CFIDS
Support Network
23732 Hillhurst Drive U-9
Laguna Niguel, California
92627

Wisconsin CEBV
Syndrome, Inc.
2141 West Fairlane Avenue
Glendale, Wisconsin 53209

In Africa

Mrs. Janine Shavell
66 Third Street
Lower-Houghton
Johannesburg

In Australia

ANZAMES
PO Box 645
Mona Vale
NSW 2103

M.E. Chronic Fatigue
Syndrome Society, Inc.
S.A. Support Group
G.P.O. Box 383
Adelaide
South Australia 5001

In Canada

M.E. Association of
Canada—Attn: Tony Gray
526 Ashfield Court
Pickering, Ontario
L1V 4W3

Mrs. K. M. Smith
PO Box 298
Kleinburg
Ontario L0J 1C0

In Europe

Marion Lescrauwaet
1106 DP Wamelplien 16
Amsterdam
The Netherlands

Ellen Piro
Gullerasveien 14B
0386 Oslo 3,
Norway

In New Zealand

ANZAMES
PO Box 35/429
Browns Bay
Auckland 10

In the United Kingdom

Myalgic Encephalomyelitis
Association
PO Box 8
Stanford le Hope
Essex SS17 8EX
(Telephone: 0375 642466)

M.E. Action Campaign
PO Box 1126
London
W3 ORY

About the Author

Steve Wilkinson writes from personal experience. In 1986 he contracted CFS, although it was not diagnosed as such for many months.

Always a strong advocate of self-help, he has managed, through the use of various alternative therapies, to restore his health to the extent that he is now largely able to live and work normally.

He works from his home in London as a writer and a healer, and he continues to conduct research with other sufferers into ways in which CFS can be alleviated.

INDEX